Endocarditis - Diagnosis and Treatment

Edited by Peter Magnusson, Payam Behzadi, Jo Ann LeQuang and Joseph V. Pergolizzi

Published in London, United Kingdom

Endocarditis - Diagnosis and Treatment
http://dx.doi.org/10.5772/intechopen.100932
Edited by Peter Magnusson, Payam Behzadi, Jo Ann LeQuang and Joseph V. Pergolizzi

Contributors
Dario Buioni, Paolo Nardi, Calogera Pisano, Claudia Altieri, Giovanni Ruvolo, Nicolas Dürrleman, Walid Ben Ali, Olina Dagher, Nils Perrin, Nancy Poirier, Naomi Nakagawa, Sudeep Das De, Sanjeet Singh Avtaar Singh, Ahmed Al-Adhami, Nawwar Al-Attar, Erin Barnes, Julia Cook

First published in London, United Kingdom, 2023 by IntechOpen
IntechOpen is the global imprint of INTECHOPEN LIMITED, registered in England and Wales, registration number: 11086078, 5 Princes Gate Court, London, SW7 2QJ, United Kingdom

British Library Cataloguing-in-Publication Data
A catalogue record for this book is available from the British Library

Additional hard and PDF copies can be obtained from orders@intechopen.com

Endocarditis - Diagnosis and Treatment
Edited by Peter Magnusson, Payam Behzadi, Jo Ann LeQuang and Joseph V. Pergolizzi
p. cm.
Print ISBN 978-1-80356-740-2
Online ISBN 978-1-80356-741-9
eBook (PDF) ISBN 978-1-80356-742-6

For EU product safety concerns:
IN TECH d.o.o., Prolaz Marije Krucifikse Kozulić 3, 51000 Rijeka, Croatia,
info@intechopen.com or visit our website at intechopen.com.

Meet the editors

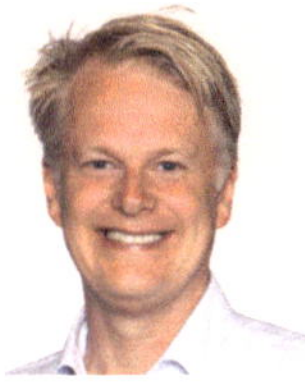

Peter Magnusson, MD, Ph.D., FESC, is a cardiologist and university lecturer. He received his MD from Lund University and Ph.D. from Karolinska Institute, Sweden. Dr. Magnusson has a broad interest in cardiovascular research, especially in structural heart disease with special emphasis on hypertrophic cardiomyopathy, heart failure, arrhythmia, device therapy, and diabetes mellitus. His research methods include both quantitative and qualitative approaches with applications to diverse study designs. He is eager to learn more and develop integration between health care and digital implementation tools. He is affiliated with the Medical School at Örebro University, Sweden. Teaching and supervision are cornerstones of his passion for disseminating knowledge.

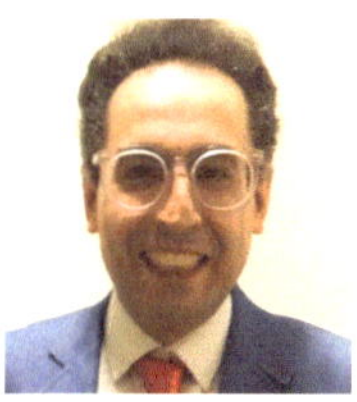

Dr. Payam Behzadi has been a faculty member at the Department of Microbiology, College of Basic Sciences, Shahr-e-Qods Branch, Islamic Azad University, Iran, since 2004. He has a BSc and MSc in Microbiology and a Ph.D. in Molecular Biology. He is currently an assistant professor at Islamic Azad University. He has authored and edited twenty-five books and book chapters and more than ninety-five original and review articles. His scientific research interests include urinary tract infections, antibiotics, bioinformatics, genetics, gene profiling, molecular biology, and cellular and molecular immunology. Dr. Behzadi trains as an ice skater in his free time.

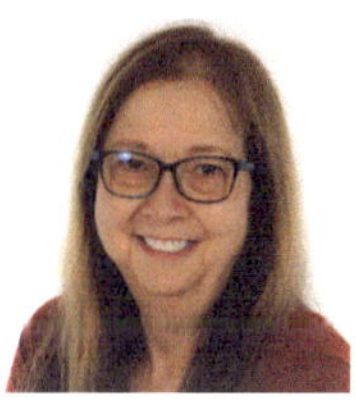

Jo Ann LeQuang, MPH, has published extensively in peer-reviewed journals on topics of critical care, perioperative care, pain management, and cardiology. She has published more than forty journal articles as well as several book chapters. In 2017, she won the Unsung Heroes Award for her advocacy for chronic pain patients

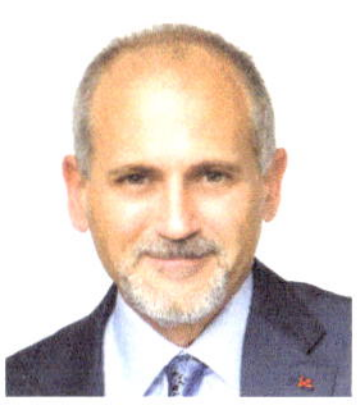

Dr. Joseph V. Pergolizzi, Jr., MD, MBA, is an internationally recognized thought leader in internal, perioperative, and pain medicine, as well as critical and palliative care, pharmacology, drug development, and regulatory affairs. He is highly published in top-tier journals.

Contents

Preface

Infective endocarditis is associated with severe morbidity and mortality. Its incidence is increasing due to an ageing population and groups at risk. Although symptoms often are unspecified, high awareness of the disease can lead to prompt diagnosis without delay, which has historically been the case. Echocardiography, including the transesophageal approach, is the first-line imaging technique for infective endocarditis. Suspicion of the condition warrants consideration of laboratory findings and history taking as well. The increasing number of patients with cardiac implants poses a certain risk. The definite diagnosis of endocarditis implies long-term antibiotics and hospitalization. Fortunately, an out-patient regimen has been advocated under certain circumstances. A tailored approach is warranted to optimize the management of suspected and confirmed endocarditis. The management of infective endocarditis is challenging and involves interaction between members from different specialists and re-evaluations. This book covers aspects of the modern, evidence-based approach to the care of endocarditis patients.

Peter Magnusson MD, Ph.D., FESC
Faculty of Medicine and Health,
School of Medical Sciences,
Örebro University,
Örebro, Sweden

Centre for Clinical Research,
Region Dalarna,
Falun, Sweden

Dr. Payam Behzadi
Department of Microbiology,
College of Basic Sciences,
Shahr-e-Qods Branch,
Islamic Azad University,
Teheran, Iran

Jo Ann LeQuang and Joseph V. Pergolizzi
NEMA Research, Inc.,
Naples, Florida, United States of America

Chapter 1

Introductory Chapter: Endocarditis – Diagnosis and Treatment

Peter Magnusson, Jo Ann LeQuang and Joseph V. Pergolizzi

1. Introduction

1.1 Endocarditis at a glance

Infective endocarditis (IE) is a major health challenge. The incidence is approximately 14 cases (1 death) per 100,000 individuals [1]. The rising numbers of IE are due to the increased population at risk, but increased awareness and availability of diagnostic tools also accounts for higher rates of diagnosed IE. Echocardiography is the cornerstone among diagnostic tools, while computerized tomography and nuclear imaging techniques have sharpened diagnostic accuracy. In patients with cardiac devices such as pacemakers and among prosthetic valve patients, modern imaging techniques are especially helpful.

The complex interplay between several conditions can lead to IE. If a surface is colonized by a pathogen *via* the bloodstream and the immunological response is ineffective, this may lead to IE. The entry of the pathogen can be skin, mouth, gastrointestinal, and urogenital as well as intravenous drugs, vascular access, or catheterization and surgical techniques. Unfortunately, antibiotic prophylaxis lacks convincing evidence. Although procedure-related antibiotics may reduce bacteremia, it may not result in the reduction of IE in general. High-risk individuals undergoing dental procedures seem to have benefited from prophylactic antibiotics according to recent data [2, 3]. Current guidelines recommend antibiotics prophylactically in four groups: previous IE and those with prosthetic valves, congenital heart disease, or ventricular assist devices [4].

For high-risk patients undergoing dental procedures, manipulating the gingiva or scaling of the root canal is recommended. Typically, streptococci should be covered; amoxicillin or cephalexin is a preferred regimen. Non-dental procedures may be associated with IE among high-risk individuals, but data are very limited still. Current guidelines have changed from no recommendation toward possible use. In cardiac or cardiovascular interventions, perioperative antibiotics are recommended. In addition, patient education regarding adequate dental and skin hygiene is crucial. Being mindful about risk groups and providing them with written educational information is advisable.

Imaging is an essential part of the diagnostic workup. Transthoracic echocardiography and transesophageal echocardiography are initial steps and often conclusive. Even though these tools are widely accessible, the quality may differ. Vegetation characteristics and size will guide therapeutic decisions. Perivalvular complications include abscess, pseudoaneurysm, valve instability, fistulas, and perforations of valves. Computerized tomography provides additional information regarding perivalvular complications. Moreover, detection of distant lesions and sources of emboli can be facilitated by computerized tomography. Magnetic resonance imaging has less spatial resolution than computerized tomography but is helpful in the detection of neurological complications in the brain of spinal cord. Position emission tomography shows high sensitivity and specificity (both more than 80%) [5].

The definitions of IE have been revised. The major criteria are blood cultures positive for IE (typical microbes from two cultures) and confirmatory imaging (echocardiography, computerized tomography, and positron emission tomography). Minor criteria are predisposing conditions, fever higher than 38 C, embolic events with vascular disseminations, immunological phenomena, and microbiological evidence. A definite diagnosis of IE requires two major criteria, or one major and three minor, or five minor criteria. A possible diagnosis is defined as one major and at least one minor or three minor without a major criteria.

Effective antibiotic therapy in IE is important for successful treatment. Typically, the bactericidal approach is beneficial. Aminoglycosides are combined with cell membrane inhibitors but may cause side effects. Often 2–6 weeks in non-valvular cases is standard treatment, whereas 6 weeks or even longer periods are used when prosthetic valves are affected. Traditionally, intravenous treatment has been advocated. However, an oral regimen after and initial phase of intravenous therapy can be used in about a fifth of the IE patients [6].

Staphylococcus aureus is the main culprit in acute and fulminant IE. Coagulase negative streptococci cause protacted valve affections [7]. Prosthetic valve endocarditis confers a high risk of death; about half of patients will die [8]. Many of these patients need surgery. Methicillin-resistant S-aureus (MRSA) is resistant to many antibiotics. Fungi are occasionally seen, most often among immunosuppressive patients, and is associated with poor outcomes.

Patients with IE have extended hospital stays that can be reduced by outpatient intravenous or oral antibiotic treatment. It is necessary to exclude patients with abscesses, heart failure, septic emboli, and stroke. The course should be stable.

Open-heart surgery is essential in some patients and results in 20% improved survival [9]. The main groups of surgical candidates are patients with acute heart failure, uncontrolled infection, and those at increased risk of septic embolization. The procedure is indicated within hours in some groups, within a few days in others, or during the hospital stay in yet another group. If antibiotics are effective, valve replacement follows the same guidelines as elective valve replacement [4].

Neurological complications can be the first manifestation of IE, or these complications may occur during treatment. Unexplained fever in conjunction with symptoms of stroke should raise the suspicion of IE with embolization. Symptomatic cerebrovascular complications occur in one third of IE patients, and four-fifths have silent neurological effects. Stroke associated with IE carries an increased risk of mortality.

Cardiac rhythm disturbances may complicate the manifestation of IE. The anatomical proximity of the valves and the conduction system makes the atrioventricular node vulnerable. Paravalvular abscess or aortic valve manifestations are more likely to be associated with severe bradycardia. Bradycardia may be caused by the spread of the infection or even by the surgery itself and may be severe enough to necessitate pacemaker implantation.

An emerging group of IE patients has transcatheter aortic valve endocarditis. The risk of IE is similar to the risk of those with surgical prostheses. The majority is elderly with less typical symptoms; for example, fever may be absent.

Cardiac devices, pacemakers, and implantable defibrillators are susceptible to infections. These patients present with fever, embolic events, and signs of pocket infections. Careful evaluations using echocardiography as well as positron emission tomography may be useful. The treatment involves early and complete removal of the entire system. This procedure should be carried out at experienced centers.

Endocarditis is a severe diagnosis and involves decision-making among specialities. Uncomplicated cases may be managed at the local level, depending on the size of the hospital. In more complicated cases, the patient should be transferred to a hospital with expertise in thoracic surgery.

Author details

Peter Magnusson[1,2]*, Jo Ann LeQuang[3] and Joseph V. Pergolizzi[3]

1 Faculty of Medicine and Health, School of Medical Sciences, Örebro University, Örebro, Sweden

2 Center for Clinical Research, Falun, Sweden

3 NEMA Research, Inc., Naples, Florida, United States of America

*Address all correspondence to: peter_michael_magnusson@hotmail.com

References

[1] Momtazmanesh S, Saeedi Moghaddam S, Malakan Rad E, Azadnajafabad S, Ebrahimi N, Mohammadi E, et al. Global, regional, and national burden and quality of care index of endocarditis: The global burden of disease study 1990-2019. European Journal of Preventive Cardiology. 2022;**29**:1287-1297

[2] Thornhill MH, Crum A, Campbell R, Stone T, Lee EC, Bradburn M, et al. Temporal association between invasive procedures and infective endocarditis. Heart. 2023;**109**:223-231

[3] Thornhill MH, Gibson TB, Yoon F, Dayer MJ, Prendergast BD, Lockhart PB, et al. Antibiotic prophylaxis against infective endocarditis before invasive dental procedures. Journal of the American College of Cardiology. 2022;**80**:1029-1041

[4] Delgado V, Marsan N, Waha S, Bonaros N, Brida M, Burri H, et al. ESC guidelines for the management of endocarditis: Developed by the task force on the management of endocarditis of the European Society of Cardiology (ESC) endorsed by the European Association for Cardio-Thoracic Surgery (EACTS) and the European Association of Nuclear Medicine (EANM). European Heart Journal. 2023:ehad193

[5] Holcman K, Szot W, Rubis P, Lesniak-Sobelga A, Hlawaty M, Wisniowska-Smialek S, et al. 99mTc-HMPAO-labeled leukocyte SPECT/CT and transthoracic echocardiography diagnostic value in infective endocarditis. The International Journal of Cardiovascular Imaging. 2019;**35**:749-758

[6] Iversen K, Ihlemann N, Gill SU, Madsen T, Elming H, Jensen KT, et al. Partial oral versus intravenous antibiotic treatment of endocarditis. The New England Journal of Medicine. 2019;**380**:415-424

[7] Sandoe JA, Kerr KG, Reynolds GW, Jain S. Staphylococcus capitis endocarditis: Two cases and review of the literature. Heart. 1999;**82**:e1

[8] Fernandez-Hidalgo N, Ribera A, Larrosa MN, Viedma E, Origuen J, de Alarcon A, et al. Impact of Staphylococcus aureus phenotype and genotype on the clinical characteristics and outcome of infective endocarditis. A multicentre, longitudinal, prospective, observational study. Clinical Microbiology and Infection. 2018;**24**:985-991

[9] Iung B, Doco-Lecompte T, Chocron S, Strady C, Delahaye F, Le Moing V, et al. Cardiac surgery during the acute phase of infective endocarditis: Discrepancies between European Society of Cardiology guidelines and practices. European Heart Journal. 2016;**37**:840-848

Chapter 2

Endocarditis: Cardiac Surgery Treatment/A Thrilling Challenge in Cardiac Surgery

Dario Buioni, Paolo Nardi, Claudia Altieri, Calogera Pisano and Giovanni Ruvolo

Abstract

Infective endocarditis is a rare but life-threatening disease that has a major impact on healthcare resources. It is heterogeneous in etiology, clinical manifestations, and course. The timing of surgery remains a topic of debate. Some authors promote an early surgical approach to improve the outcomes. There are different points of view between American and European guidelines regarding the relative priority of surgery over medical treatment. Anyway, multidisciplinary teams and multimodality strategies are advocated in order to optimize the treatment according to the individual needs of the patients. The early surgical approach may represent a valuable treatment option for high-risk patients. In this chapter, we discuss the latest evidence on surgical approaches, potential pitfalls, and the controversial issues in the contemporary practice of infective endocarditis.

Keywords: complicated infective endocariditis, cardiac device, surgical reconstruction, echocardiography imaging, prosthetic heart valve

1. Introduction

Infective endocarditis (IE) is a rare but severe cause of sepsis that consumes considerable healthcare resources and requires multidisciplinary approach. It affects 3–10 per 100,000 per year in the population, and the incidence seems to be slightly increasing [1]. Therefore, up to 40–50% of affected patients require valve surgery during the clinical course, with overall mortality remaining around 20–25% per year in most published series. First described by Lazare Riviere in the seventeenth century, but William Osler better characterized the clinical manifestations [2]. Given its complexity, the management of infective endocarditis requires the close collaboration of multidisciplinary approach, Endocarditis Team, mandatory for the appropriate initial treatment. It is generally agreed that those decisions on both the indication and timing of surgical intervention should be determined by multi-specialists with expertise in cardiology, imaging, cardiac surgery, infectious disease, and neurology [3]. Approximately 50% of patients will require early surgery, but there are concerns that performing the procedure during an active infection, before the valve is completely sterilized, may lead to an increase in post-operative complications. Despite the rapid diagnosis and early intervention, 1-year mortality associated with erectile dysfunction has not improved in recent decades. Infectious endocarditis on prosthetic material after percutaneous procedures represent over 25% of all cases and include electronic implantable cardiac device (CIED), TAVR transcatheter aortic valve replacement, non-electronic devices (percutaneous occluder), cases of which are on the rise and create unique clinical challenges [4]. Interventions are characterized by a high risk of mortality. The use of surgery has gained a phase in the treatment of IE, and it is expanding. Current guidelines are cautious in board indication of surgery in aggressive left-sided endocarditis [5]. Early surgery is highly recommended in patients with IE with signs of congestive heart failure, while surgery to prevent systemic embolism remains debated. Indeed, main concern for patients with large vegetation high-risk embolism [6]. In these cases, the early surgery approach with complete excision of infected tissue and valve repair has been achieved in high-volume centers with low mortality, suggesting the benefit of early surgical management [7]. Concerns remain regarding the technical challenge of surgery in the active infection and inflammatory responses. The 2015 American College of Cardiology-American Heart Association (ACC-AHA) and European Society of Cardiology guidelines on the use of early surgery have different approaches and non-univocal recommendation [8]. There is a difference in the assessment of endocarditis between the European and American guidelines that can guide the decision-making aspect. For the ESC guidelines, distinguish emergency surgery (performed within 24 h), urgent surgery (within a few days), and elective surgery (after 1–2 weeks of antibiotic therapy), with an urgent basis for the majority of cases [9–11]. AHA guidelines define early surgery as during initial hospitalization and before completion of a full course of antibiotics. At the moment, there are no randomized studies that can help us reach the best conditions for the surgery and, therefore, the right times. Crucial for the best surgical outcome, to perform it at the right time, especially in patients with prosthetic valve endocarditis, which occurs in 3–6% of patients within 5 years of surgery and is characterized by high morbidity and mortality. Many patients considered at intermediate to high risk or inoperable that have undergone TAVR are also susceptible to IE on these prostheses [12, 13]. There are well-known patients subset that are at higher risk due to anatomical features of valve heart disease and coexistent comorbidities, with more than 10% of patients considered to be at too high risk for surgery [14].

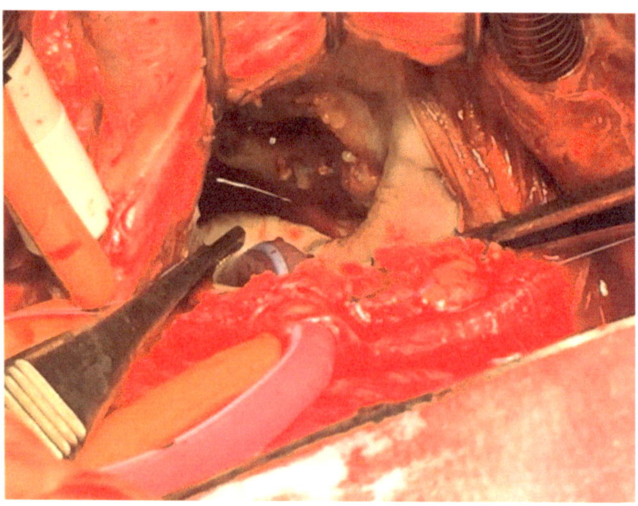

Figure 1.
Mitral annulus endocarditis.

Although surgical techniques, prosthetic models, anesthesiology, and infectiology approaches have constantly improved over the last years, increased higher-risk cases may affect operative success, in terms of higher mortality. Finally, surgery approach; valve conservation is especially important in less developed populations where compliance with medical therapy, especially anticoagulation, is poor, and bioprostheses are prone to early degeneration in young patients. Repair of the aortic valve is generally only applied to minor lesions, such as localized perforations of the cusps and vegetations that do not significantly alter the valve structure. In contrast, there is a wider scope for conservation of the mitral valve (MV); several studies have confirmed the feasibility of MV repair in the healed and active phase of IE and have shown better long-term results in comparison with valve replacement. Several authors used a minimally invasive or endoscopic approach. In this chapter, we will discuss the surgeon's point of view and can be given answers regarding the best strategy to be adopted in the early treatment of IE (**Figure 1**).

2. Epidemiology

In the past, rheumatic heart disease was a predisposing condition, but is nowadays less commonly detected among cases of infective endocarditis, although the importance of such predisposing conditions persists in low-income countries [15]. Therefore to know the real patient age, comorbidities, place of acquisition, type of endocarditis, microbiological data, and mortality rate worldwide. Cases associated with intravenous drug use have decreased, but dramatic increase in North America and in some Eastern European countries [16]. In high-income countries, cases are increasing for degenerative valve disease, intracardiac devices, indwelling catheters, and immunosuppression [17, 18]. This explains why the latest analyses of the demographic of endocarditis cases show a trend toward nosocomial characteristics, elderly patients, staphylococcal, enterococcal cases, and the involvement of prosthetic valves and cardiovascular implantable electronic devices (CIEDs). Other etiologies: 2–5% can be produced by Gram-negative bacilli (HACEK group [19]). Fungal endocarditis accounts for less than 2% of cases, mainly caused by yeasts of the genus *Candida spp* and rarely by other filamentous fungal yeasts [20]. A variable proportion (up to 10–20% of cases) without documented etiology is considered "culture-negative endocarditis" mostly as a consequence of prior administration of antibiotics or caused either by slow-growing microorganisms or from intracellular bacteria that are difficult to cultivate (e.g., *Chlamydophila spp.*, *Bartonella spp.*, *Tropheryma whipplei*). *Staphylococcus aureus* is the most frequently isolated pathogen in high-income countries with a reported percentage of 30% of cases. Habib et al. In the EURO-ENDO registry, from 1 January 2016 to 31 March 2018, centers were asked to include consecutive patients aged greater than 18 years who presented with IE during a 1-year period [21]. A total of 156 centers from 40 countries included 3116 cases of IE, representing an average of 20.19 patients per center per year offers a unique opportunity to assess the current characteristics of IE in Europe [22]. It allows us to consider clinical presentation, microbiology, complications, management, and prognosis. Several countries outside Europe also participated in this study, allowing the analysis of IE on the basis of geographical and socioeconomic factors. It will allow a comparison with the EuroHeart survey [23, 24]. The main messages emerging from EURO ENDO: IE most frequently affects men around 60 years of age; prosthetic valve infective endocarditis (PVIE), CIED, nosocomial, staphylococcal, and enterococcal endocarditis are more frequent. Sepsis and septic shock are severe complications that may arise from any type of infection, which can eventually lead to a multiorgan failure. It appears to be associated with particularly virulent microorganisms such as *S. aureus* and beta-hemolytic Streptococci. Indeed, due to their invasive and destructive effects on the affected anatomical structures, these bacteria can seed distant septic metastases. The extraction of exotoxins that can act as superantigens, which overactivate the immune system. The systemic inflammation that is consequently triggered has an important hemodynamic impact, with endothelial dysfunction and a drop in vascular resistance. This serious situation explains why the presence of septic shock is associated with an increase in the risk of mortality. IE develops in three stages: bacteremia, adhesion, and colonization. In bacteremia, bacteria enter the bloodstream via the mouth, gastrointestinal, and urinary tracts, or the skin, through venous catheters or after an invasive medical or surgical procedure. Adhesion: whereas the normal endothelial lining of the heart is resistant to bacterial adhesion, bacteria are able to adhere to abnormal or damaged endothelium via surface adhesins. These proteins mediate attachment to extracellular host matrix proteins, facilitated by fibrin and platelet microthrombi. Bacterial adhesion gives rise to colonization; cycles of bacterial proliferation occur in addition to thrombosis, monocyte recruitment, and inflammation, leading to formation of mature vegetation. Many of the microorganisms produce biofilms that protect bacteria host immune defenses, impede antimicrobial efficacy, and hide resistant persister organisms. Biofilm is an important determinant of virulence in staphylococcal device-related infections. In general, three blood culture series detect the presence of pathogens in 96–98% of bacteremia who have not yet started antibiotic therapy, in coagulase-negative Staphylococci. The blood culture does not need to be done at the febrile peak because the presence of the pathogen is not related to the extent of the fever. It's possible that no pathogen growth from blood cultures delays diagnosis, which, is reported in up to 10% of cases. Fungal endocarditis usually caused by Candida or Aspergillus, is very aggressive and often fatal because it occurs in the immunosuppressed patient or after cardiac surgery, mainly in prosthetic valve recipients. After surgery can help in the microbiological diagnosis through the use

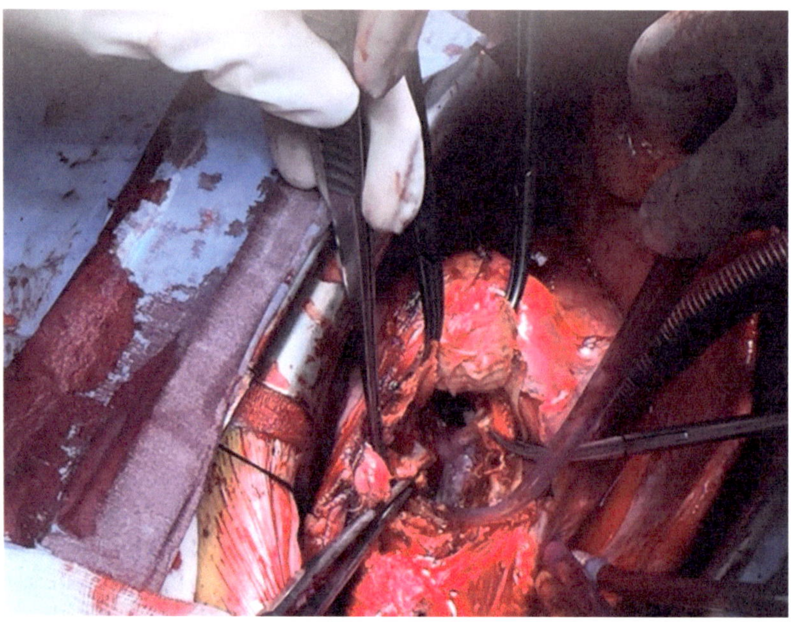

Figure 2.
Prosthesis aortic valve infection.

of complementary molecular techniques such as a polymerase chain reaction for pathogen DNA (PCR). Particularly useful in patients that received antibiotics, as bacterial DNA often persists even for non-cultivable pathogens (e.g. *T. whipplei*). PCR often carries the risk of false positive results due to contamination of the sample. New techniques combining PCR and mass spectrometry promise direct characterization of bacteria in peripheral blood or valvular tissue. The infection that occurs on cardiac devices is sustained by reactive inflammatory and thrombotic phenomena (**Figure 2**).

3. Diagnosis

The diagnosis of IE is based on clinical, microbiological, and imaging data, as specified by the modified Duke criteria. Clinical features of infective endocarditis remains a critical feature in diagnosis, primarily for subacute and chronic forms. For diagnosis the information proposed by blood cultures, and different imaging can accurately define anatomical aspects such as vegetation or other complications [25].

4. Imaging

Transthoracic echocardiography (TTE) is the main method in the diagnosis of endocarditis; remains cornerstone of imaging and is rapid, straightforward, and may diagnostic. TTE is the recommended initial modality of choice for both native or prosthetic valve infective endocarditis (TTE) varying sensitivity rates for valvular and paravalvular abnormalities such as vegetations, new regurgitation, or dehiscence of a prosthetic valve perforations, abscesses, and fistulae. Transesophageal echocardiography TEE is indicated when TTE is positive or nondiagnostic, when complications are suspected, or when intracardiac device leads are present. This technique can also differentiate vegetations from thrombi and can be used in surgical planning. A growing interest in the use of cardiac computed tomography (CT) [26]. CT shows anatomical correlation, especially when diagnosing a perivalvular abscess of the aortomitral intervalvular fibrous body and structures surrounding the aortic root. Cardiac CT is frequently used to preoperatively assess the presence of coronary artery disease in aortic endocarditis where performing a coronary angiography carries a prohibitively high risk of dislodging of vegetation. In early diagnosis, excellent results are obtained in measuring biological activity by emission of 18 F-fluorodeoxyglucose positron/computed tomography (FDG-PET/CT) and CT/CT with emission of single photons of radiolabelled white blood cells (WBC-SPECT/CT). These investigation methods have been recommended by the European Society of Cardiology in patients with suspected endocarditis on valves implanted for more than 3 months, whose positive value has been included as the main criterion for the diagnosis of the germ and therefore of device-related endocarditis [27]. Several studies on patients with suspected PVE have demonstrated an important diagnostic value of FDG-PET/CT and WBC-SPECT/CT and suggest that two imaging techniques can be used in a stepwise fashion when evaluating the presence of endocarditis. FDG-PET/CT should be used first, for higher sensitivity and if the results are not conclusive, WBC-SPECT/CT may be performed. Controversy remains on the use in patients with aortic root grafts with a prosthetic valve, since a high rate of false positives. In the diagnosis of NVE, the role of FDG-PET/CT has not been fully established and may be limited when endocarditis is strongly suspected but the DUKE criteria are not met [28]. Brain CT is often used when neurological symptoms are present, and magnetic resonance imaging (MRI) has better sensitivity in defining lesions. Routine cerebral RMI identifies abnormalities in 80% of patients. Routine cross-sectional imaging of the brain, chest, spine, spleen, liver, and kidneys has not demonstrated a clear utility, but evidence of embolism by cross-sectional imaging is a novel minor diagnostic criterion in the ESC 2015 guidelines.

5. Surgery approach

The objectives of surgery are as follows: remove possible sources of embolism; remove both infected tissue and foreign material; restore cardiac integrity, close any cavities; and often restore both the aortic mitral junction and the left ventricular outflow tract. Many surgical techniques have been used or invented both full sternotomy and minimally invasive approaches, but a clear long-term advantage of one technique has yet to be proven [29, 30]. Surgery is currently performed in 50–60% of patients, and 6-month survival rates are >80%. Current indications for surgery, as defined in the AHA and ESC guidelines. The optimal timing of surgical intervention is also contentious [31]. Delaying surgery may allow a high risk of disease progression with valve destruction, abscess formation, heart block, embolic complications, and even death [32]. Early surgery differs significantly between European and U.S. guidelines. The most common indication to perform early operation in the IE is the development of heart failure. Severe valve regurgitation, even among asymptomatic patients, imposes a volume load on the left ventricle, which results in ventricular dysfunction for dilatation or hypertrophy and heart failure. In mitral valve regurgitation, the elevation of left atrial pressure leads to left atrial enlargement, atrial fibrillation, and pulmonary congestion. In patients who had not received emergency surgery, the outcomes are nefarious because of the progression to cardiogenic shock. The large vegetation that comprises the functionality of the entire valve can have a faster deterioration with the progression of hemodynamic instability. Once the diagnosis of IE has been ascertained and the indication for surgery is formulated, there currently appears to be no demonstrated benefit in delaying surgery. The choice to perform ED surgery in the first few hours or with a 48-hour delay depends on the evaluation of the endocarditis team but above all on the patient's clinic. Mortality is low in centers of excellence with high-level experience in the management of complex patients, although very often, especially in complex or repetitive cases, it is not possible to standardize surgical techniques.

Author details

Dario Buioni*, Paolo Nardi, Claudia Altieri, Calogera Pisano and Giovanni Ruvolo
Cardiac Surgery Unit, Tor Vergata University Hospital, Rome, Italy

*Address all correspondence to: docyuk@libero.it

References

[1] Miro JM, Ambrosioni J. Infective endocarditis: An ongoing global challenge. European Heart Journal. 2019;**40**(39):3233-3236. DOI: 10.1093/eurheartj/ehz694

[2] Benedicto A, Domínguez L. Endocarditis and cardiac device infections. In: Firstenberg MS, Lakshmanadoss U, editors. Advanced Concepts in Endocarditis (Chapter 7). London, UK: IntechOpen; 2021. DOI: 10.5772/intechopen.96909

[3] Cahill T, Baddour L, Habib G, et al. Challenges in infective endocarditis. Journal of the American College of Cardiology. 2017;**69**(3):325-344. DOI: 10.1016/j.jacc.2016.10.066

[4] Mack M, Lancellotti P, et al. Early surgery in infective endocarditis. Journal of the American College of Cardiology. 2020;**76**(1):41-42. DOI: 10.1016/j.jacc.2020.05.049

[5] Gomes A, Jainandunsing JS, van Assen S, van Geel PP, Sinha B, Gelsomino S, et al. A standardized approach to treat complex aortic valve endocarditis: A case series. Journal of Cardiothoracic Surgery. 2018;**13**(1):32. DOI: 10.1186/s13019-018-0715-8

[6] Ivanovic B, Trifunovic D, Matic S, Petrovic J, Sacic D, Tadic M. Prosthetic valve endocarditis—A trouble or a challenge? Journal of Cardiology. 2019;**73**(2):126-133. DOI: 10.1016/j.jjcc.2018.08.007. Epub 2018 Oct 30

[7] Salem M, Friedrich C, Saad M, Frank D, Salem M, Puehler T, et al. Active infective native and prosthetic valve endocarditis: Short- and long-term outcomes of patients after surgical treatment. Journal of Clinical Medicine. 2021;**10**(9):1868. DOI: 10.3390/jcm10091868

[8] Habib G, Lancellotti P, Antunes MJ, Bongiorni MG, Casalta J-P, Del Zotti F, et al. Endorsed by: European Association for Cardio-Thoracic Surgery (EACTS), the European Association of Nuclear Medicine (EANM). European Heart Journal. 2015;**36**(44):3075-3128. DOI: 10.1093/eurheartj/ehv319

[9] Nishimura A, Otto CM, Bonow RO, Carabello BA, Erwin JP 3rd, Fleisher LA, et al. 2017 AHA/ACC focused update of the 2014 AHA/ACC guideline for the management of patients with valvular heart disease: A report of the American College of Cardiology/American Heart Association task force on clinical practice guidelines. Circulation. 2017;**135**:e1159-e1195. DOI: 10.1161/CIR.0000000000000503

[10] Flynn CD, Curran NP, Chan S, Zegri-Reiriz I, Tauron M, Tian DH, et al. Systematic review and meta-analysis of surgical outcomes comparing mechanical valve replacement and bioprosthetic valve replacement in infective endocarditis. Annals of Cardiothoracic Surgery. 2019;**8**(6):587-599. DOI: 10.21037/acs.2019.10.03

[11] Habib G, Erba PA, Iung B, Donal E, Cosyns B, Laroche C, et al. Clinical presentation, aetiology and outcome of infective endocarditis. Results of the ESC-EORP EURO-ENDO (European infective endocarditis) registry: A prospective cohort study. European Heart Journal. 2019;**40**(39):3222-3232. DOI: 10.1093/eurheartj/ehz620. Erratum in: European Heart Journal 2020;41(22):2091

[12] Van Vlasselaer A et al. Native aortic versus mitral valve infective endocarditis:

A nationwide registry study. Open Heart. 2019;**6**

[13] Satriano UM, Nenna A, Spadaccio C, Pollari F, Fischlein T, Chello M, et al. Guidelines on prosthetic heart valve management in infective endocarditis: A narrative review comparing American Heart Association/American College of Cardiology and European Society of cardiology guidelines. Annals of Translational Medicine. 2020;**8**(23):1625. DOI: 10.21037/atm-20-5134

[14] Bin Abdulhak AA, Qazi AH, Tleyjeh IM. Workup and management of native and prosthetic valve endocarditis. Current Treatment Options in Cardiovascular Medicine. 2018;**20**(9):73. DOI: 10.1007/s11936-018-0668-1

[15] Chan V. When should infective endocarditis be treated with early surgical intervention? The Canadian Journal of Cardiology. 2018;**34**(9):1110-1111. DOI: 10.1016/j.cjca.2018.06.013. Epub 2018 Jun 30

[16] Olmos C, Vilacosta I, Habib G, Maroto L, Fernández C, López J, et al. Risk score for cardiac surgery in active left-sided infective endocarditis. Heart. 2017;**103**(18):1435-1442. DOI: 10.1136/heartjnl-2016-311093. Epub 2017 Apr 21

[17] Farag M, Borst T, Sabashnikov A, Zeriouh M, Schmack B, Arif R, et al. Surgery for infective endocarditis: Outcomes and predictors of mortality in 360 consecutive patients. Medical Science Monitor. 2017;**23**:3617-3626. DOI: 10.12659/MSM.902340

[18] Khan A, Aslam A, Satti KN, Ashiq S. Infective endocarditis post-transcatheter aortic valve implantation (TAVI), microbiological profile and clinical outcomes: A systematic review. PLoS One. 2020;**15**(1):e0225077. DOI: 10.1371/journal.pone.0225077

[19] Bjursten H, Rasmussen M, Nozohoor S, Götberg M, Olaison L, Rück A, et al. Infective endocarditis after transcatheter aortic valve implantation: A nationwide study. European Heart Journal. 2019;**40**(39):3263-3269. DOI: 10.1093/eurheartj/ehz588

[20] Erbel R. The new strategy in infective endocarditis: Early surgery based on early diagnosis: Are we too late when early surgery is best? Circulation. 2015;**131**(2):121-123. DOI: 10.1161/CIRCULATIONAHA.114.013872. Epub 2014 Dec 5

[21] Mastrobuoni S, Chan V, Ruel M. Early surgery for infective endocarditis. The New England Journal of Medicine. 2012;**367**(14):1365-1366; author reply 1366-7. DOI: 10.1056/NEJMc1209897

[22] Nasso G, Santarpino G, Moscarelli M, Condello I, Dell'Aquila AM, Peivandi AD, et al. Surgical treatment of valve endocarditis in high-risk patients and predictors of long-term outcomes. Scientific Reports. 2021;**11**(1):24223. DOI: 10.1038/s41598-021-03602-3

[23] Nappi F, Iervolino A, Singh SSA. The new challenge for heart endocarditis: From conventional prosthesis to new devices and platforms for the treatment of structural heart disease. BioMed Research International. 2021;**2021**:7302165. DOI: 10.1155/2021/7302165

[24] Cuervo G, Escrihuela-Vidal F, Gudiol C, Carratalà J. Current challenges in the management of infective endocarditis. Frontiers in Medicine (Lausanne). 2021;**8**:641243. DOI: 10.3389/fmed.2021.641243

[25] Gordon SM, Pettersson GB. Native-valve infective endocarditis—When does it require surgery? The New England Journal of Medicine.

2012;**366**(26):2519-2521. DOI: 10.1056/NEJMe1205453

[26] Liang F, Song B, Liu R, Yang L, Tang H, Li Y. Optimal timing for early surgery in infective endocarditis: A meta-analysis. Interactive Cardiovascular and Thoracic Surgery. 2016;**22**(3):336-345. DOI: 10.1093/icvts/ivv368. Epub 2015 Dec 17

[27] Benedetto U, Spadaccio C, Gentile F. A narrative review of early surgery versus conventional treatment for infective endocarditis: Do we have an answer? Annals of Translational Medicine. 2020;**8**(23):1626

[28] Antunes MJ. Mitral valve repair versus replacement for infective endocarditis. What is better in the "real world"? The Journal of Thoracic and Cardiovascular Surgery. 2018;**156**(4):1471-1472. DOI: 10.1016/j.jtcvs.2018.05.010. Epub 2018 May 28

[29] Zubarevich A, Zhigalov K, Osswald A, Arjomandi Rad A, Vardanyan R, Wendt D, et al. Essen-commando: How we do it. Journal of Cardiac Surgery. 2021;**36**(1):286-289. DOI: 10.1111/jocs.15140. Epub 2020 Oct 21

[30] Weltert L, Gaudino M. Commentary: Even simplified, it is still a commando operation. JTCVS Techniques. 2020;**4**:104-105. DOI: 10.1016/j.xjtc.2020.09.010

[31] Chen P, Chang C, Chuang Y, Chen I, Lin T. Modified commando procedure in complicated infective endocarditis—A case series. Journal of Cardiothoracic Surgery. 2021;**16**(1):79. DOI: 10.1186/s13019-021-01480-4

[32] Elde S, de Biasi A, Woo YJ, Burton É. A novel alternative to the commando procedure: Constructing a neo-aortic root by anchoring to the sewing ring of the replaced mitral valve. JTCVS Techniques. 2020;**4**:101-102. DOI: 10.1016/j.xjtc.2020.08.037. Epub 2020 Aug 28

Chapter 3

Tricuspid Valve Infective Endocarditis

Olina Dagher, Walid Ben Ali, Nils Perrin, Nancy Poirier and Nicolas Dürrleman

Abstract

The tricuspid valve, which has been known as the "forgotten valve", must not be ignored in infective endocarditis. Tricuspid valve infective endocarditis is a very complex condition and occurs in a complex patient population. The causative organisms are often highly virulent and patients usually have a history of intravenous drug abuse. Although the success rate of antibiotic therapy is high, certain features or complications may require surgery. Understanding the therapeutic options, the challenges of surgical intervention and the components of the patient-centered longitudinal care plan is crucial in order to minimize the risk of relapse, which is unfortunately not uncommon in these patients.

Keywords: tricuspid valve, infective endocarditis, tricuspid valve repair, tricuspid valve replacement, intravenous drug use

1. Introduction

In order to feel comfortable with tricuspid valve surgery, one has to have an excellent understanding of the peculiarities of right heart surgery. Surgical interventions on the right heart have many unique characteristics which differ significantly from those of the left heart. These must not be overlooked. Right heart surgery has a false reputation of being more "forgiving" in case of a technical error or a complication. Here are other distorted viewpoints that sometimes resurface: "If the left heart works well, the right heart follows", or "Anything can work on the right heart". Believing that surgery on the right heart is less challenging than surgery on the left heart is a perilous perception. Experience has taught us that this is far from being the case. We would even argue that it's the opposite. Right heart surgery requires additional experience and rigorous technical skills.

The right ventricle is highly compliant and is able to accommodate an important increase in preload conditions (**Figure 1**), such as in tricuspid regurgitation, even in the acute phase. The occurrence of symptomatic right heart failure under these hemodynamic circumstances will therefore be delayed compared to left heart failure secondary to acute mitral insufficiency. However, this pathophysiologic attribute can turn into a hurdle following tricuspid valve repair or replacement: the symptom recovery curve follows the same trajectory as symptom progression and correction of the tricuspid regurgitation may not yield immediate symptomatic improvements. In the meantime,

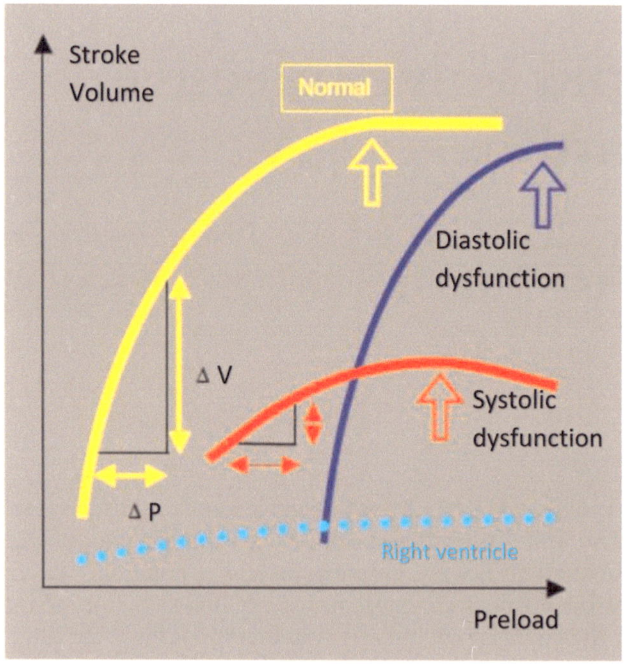

Figure 1.
Frank-Starling curve of the failing right ventricle (dotted line), which is much flatter compared to that of the failing left ventricle: Its stroke volume variation is minimal with the increase in preload.

the right heart, which is afterload-sensitive, must increase its output while facing more resistance. The right ventricle can therefore be more vulnerable than the left ventricle in certain scenarios. This concern feeds to the controversy of appropriate surgical timing for tricuspid intervention [1]. Current evidence seems to be in favor of early intervention [2]. Experts in the field of mitral valve surgery have also studied the progression of tricuspid valve disease following successful mitral valve repair [3]. They highlighted the importance of prophylactic tricuspid annuloplasty during mitral valve surgery for more severe cases of tricuspid annular dilation [3].

Myocardial protection of the right ventricle is very delicate and cross-clamping may subject the right ventricle to deleterious injuries that might not be as well tolerated as the left ventricle. In fact, intuitively, experienced cardiac surgeons will say that if right ventricular function is preserved following aortic unclamping, it indicates that myocardial protection was adequate. In case of suboptimal myocardial protection, signs of myocardial dysfunction will usually be more evident in the right ventricle. It is sometimes thought that right heart "resuscitation" can simply be achieved with replacement fluid therapy. However, the right ventricle is more sensitive to conduction and rhythm disturbances compared to the left ventricle. As mentioned previously, the right ventricle is also highly afterload-sensitive. Right ventricular afterload can be defined by pulmonary vascular resistance. This is why pulmonary hypertension should be aggressively treated perioperatively. The use of milrinone and nitric oxide to achieve afterload reduction have contributed to a significant improvement in outcomes of patients with right ventricular dysfunction. Other vasopressors and inotropes, such as vasopressin, norepinephrine, or epinephrine, can provide additional support and help to recover right heart function. These drugs are especially useful in systemic inflammatory conditions such as infective endocarditis which can be accompanied by hypotension. In addition, acutely elevated inflammatory biomarkers are a strong predictor of short-term adverse outcomes [4]. Therefore, if the patient's clinical state allows it, differing surgical intervention until peak inflammation subsides might improve prognosis.

Lastly, an important technical point to be cognizant of is the delicate tissue manipulation that is required when operating on infected right-sided structures: the latter, being more fragile at baseline compared to left-sided structures, can be easily damaged. In those circumstances, the pericardium, whether autologous or heterologous, becomes an indispensable material.

2. Anatomical characteristics of the tricuspid valve

2.1 The tricuspid valve complex

As its name suggests, the tricuspid valve is generally composed of three cusps or leaflets. The leaflets are named by the position of their annular attachment: septal, anterior and posterior. While the leaflets vary in their circumferential and area sizes, the posterior leaflet is the smallest [5]. The septal leaflet (**Figure 2**) has distinct characteristics: it has a narrow, rectangular, shape and is inserted directly into the membranous septum via many third-order chordae [6].

The subvalvular apparatus of the tricuspid valve is similar to that of the mitral valve: the presence of papillary muscles (contractile function) and chordae tendinae (elastic function) (**Figure 3**) allow for a functionally dynamic behavior [7]. The tricuspid valve apparatus includes 2 main papillary muscles (anterior and posterior), as well as a third variable and rudimentary papillary muscle (septal) [5]. The anterior papillary muscle is typically the largest and the most constant one [8]. It lends chordal support to the anterior and posterior leaflets, and, occasionally, to the moderator band [6]. The posterior papillary muscle supports the posterior and septal leaflets [6]. The four valves, including the tricuspid, lie within the fibrous skeleton of the heart (**Figure 4**). The fibrous continuity occurs through the fibrous annulus of the tricuspid valve, providing a firm support structure for the valve. However, unlike the mitral

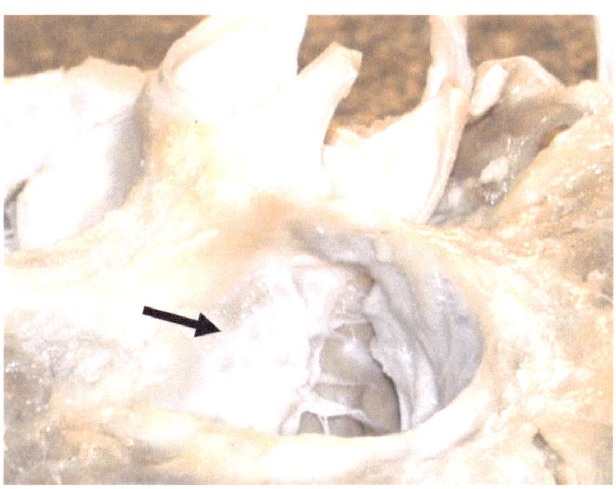

Figure 2.
Septal leaflet of the tricuspid valve (black arrow).

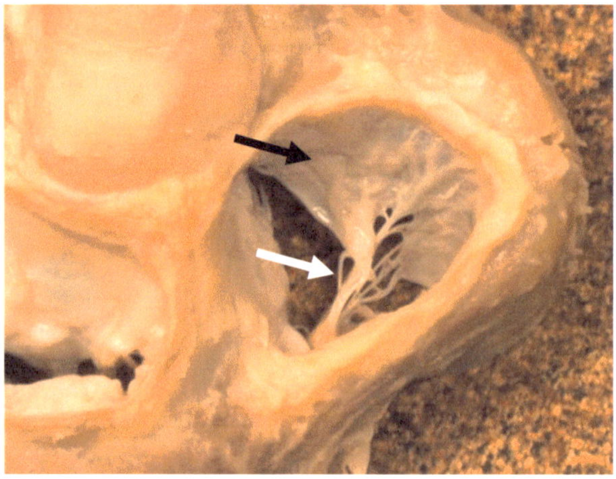

Figure 3.
Chordae tendinae (white arrow) attaching to the anterior leaflet of the tricuspid valve (black arrow).

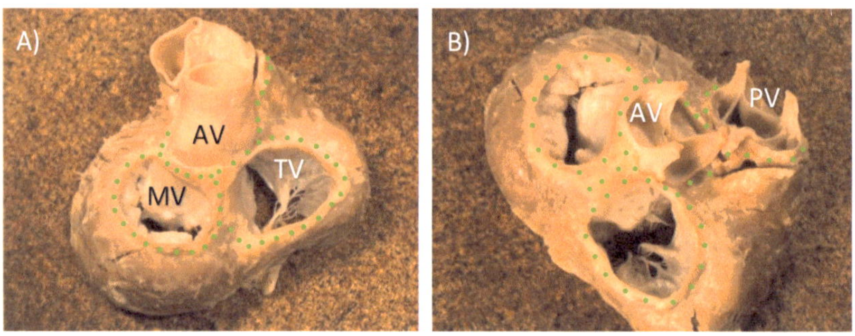

Figure 4.
A and B) fibrous cardiac skeleton (green dots) anchors the four cardiac valves. AV: Aortic valve; MV: Mitral valve; PV: Pulmonary valve; TV: Tricuspid valve.

valve, the tricuspid valve has no fibrous continuity with its corresponding semilunar valve [6]. Despite having different spatial positions and orientations within the cardiac fibrous skeleton, all four cardiac valves are anchored to that inert collagen framework. Understanding the anatomic conformation of the fibrous skeleton is crucial to understanding the structure–function relationships of each heart valve with other cardiac entities, such as heart chambers, coronary arteries or the conduction system. It then becomes intuitive to predict both the natural history of a disease and the iatrogenic complications related to its management.

2.2 Anatomical relationships of the tricuspid valve with other cardiac structures

2.2.1 Right coronary artery

The course of the right coronary artery is intimately related to the anterior and posterior leaflets of the tricuspid valve (**Figure 5**). In the setting of tricuspid valve endocarditis, bacterial invasion can spread into the tricuspid ring and form a periannular abscess. The abscess may cause an erosion of the adjacent tissues such as the coronary artery wall, resulting in coronary-cameral fistulae between the right

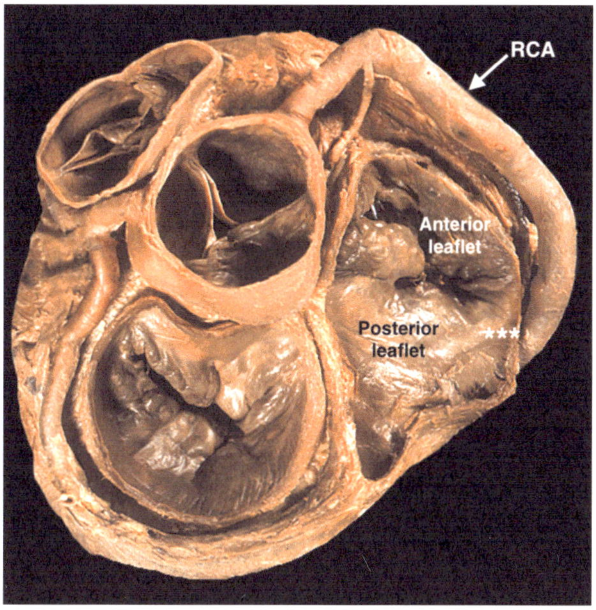

Figure 5.
Superior view of cadaveric heart valves (normal anatomy). The anterior wall of the heart is at the top of the picture and the left and right atria were removed. The coronary arteries were dissected. The right coronary artery (RCA) is in close proximity to the antero-posterior aspect of the tricuspid valve annulus (white asterisks).

coronary artery and the right atrium or the right ventricle [9]. Paradoxically, congenital anomalies of the coronary arteries are a well-recognized risk factor of infective endocarditis [10]. Septic coronary thrombosis is another rare but potential complication since infective endocarditis causes an impairment of immunothrombosis [10]. During tricuspid valve repair or replacement, iatrogenic injury to the right coronary artery (occlusion, thrombosis or dissection) can occur either directly from suturing through or around the artery, or indirectly from the tension placed on adjacent tissue and leading to a kinking mechanism once the sutures are pulled taut [11].

2.2.2 Conduction system

The tricuspid valve complex is closely associated with the conduction system and this has important implications for tricuspid valve repair and replacement.

The anatomy of the conduction system at the atrioventricular junctions has been extensively described by Anderson et al. [12, 13]. The atrioventricular node is located at the base of the septal aspect of the right atrium, just above the tricuspid valve. The bundle of His, which connects the atrioventricular node to the left and right bundle branches, is located just below the postero-superior margin of the membranous septum. The triangle of Koch serves an as an anatomic landmark for the location of the atrioventricular node. The triangle of Koch is delineated by the continuation of the Eustachian ridge as the tendon of Todaro and by the hinge of the septal leaflet of the tricuspid valve. These borders meet at the membranous septum, forming the apex of the triangle. The tendon of Todaro can be identified by gently pulling on the coronary sinus, which will reveal a linear prominence connecting the coronary sinus to the anteroseptal commissure of the tricuspid valve. The apical region of the triangle of Koch contains the atrioventricular node before it becomes a penetrating bundle, the

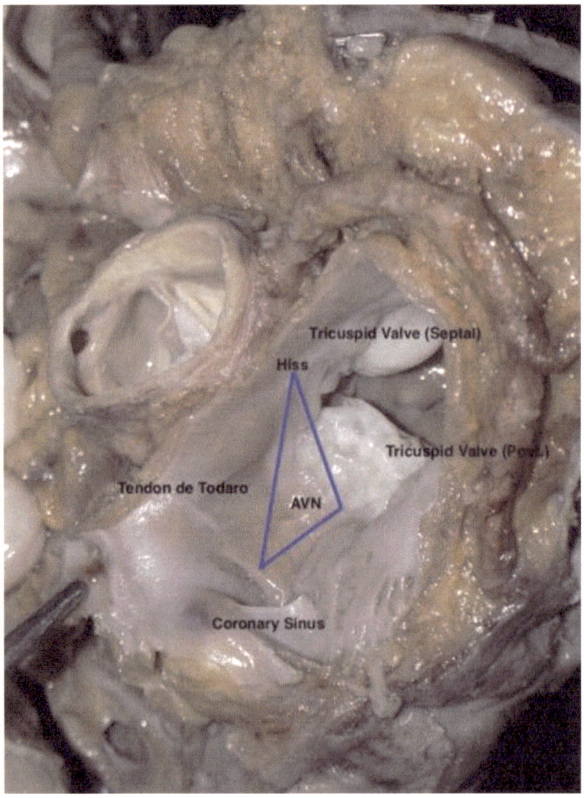

Figure 6.
Triangle of Koch (blue).

bundle of His, and enters the membranous septum at the apex (**Figure 6**). The atrioventricular conduction axis is surrounded with the insulating tissues of the central fibrous body. One should therefore keep in mind that any traumatic lesion to the conduction system around the atrioventricular junction could lead to a complete atrioventricular block, necessitating a permanent pacemaker implantation. Indeed, during tricuspid annuloplasty, the use of an open "C" ring avoids the necessity of suturing near the atrioventricular node, reducing the risks of complete heart block.

2.2.3 Left atrium

Right to left inter-atrial shunts related to tricuspid valve endocarditis and subsequent severe tricuspid regurgitation have been previously reported [14, 15]. In these cases, the regurgitant jet was being directed across an inter-atrial defect, patent foramen ovale or atrial septal defect, causing an acute right to left shunt. Depending on the magnitude of the shunt, patients can develop significant symptoms from refractory hypoxia and heart failure.

2.2.4 Right coronary sinus of Valsalva

Involvement of the right coronary sinus of Valsalva in the context of infective endocarditis is typically seen with double-valve endocarditis involving both the aortic

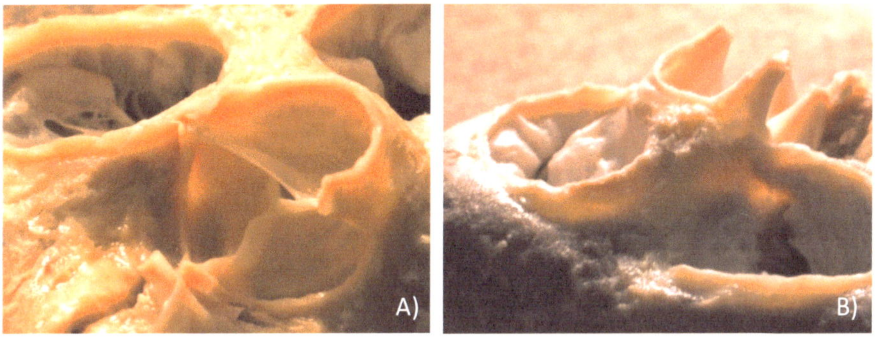

Figure 7.
Anatomic relationship between the right coronary sinus of Valsalva and the septal aspect of the tricuspid valve from the a) aortic view and B) the tricuspid view.

and the tricuspid valves [16]. The infection may originate from the aortic leaflets and invade the tricuspid valve through the periannular structures abutting the right coronary sinus of Valsalva (**Figure** 7). This should be suspected in cases of aortic valve endocarditis associated with a heart block, even after a reassuring echocardiogram that had no signs of tricuspid regurgitation. During surgical intervention, careful exploration should be undertaken to exclude the presence of a contiguous abscess. Lastly, the right coronary sinus may develop aneurysmal dilatation caused by mycotic degeneration of the arterial wall [16].

3. Preoperative evaluation

3.1 Clinical evaluation

Performing a clinical baseline assessment is important not only to allow for a coherent medical surveillance, but also to rule out a left-sided endocarditis and therefore a systemic dissemination. Any sign of left-sided or systemic infection in the context of tricuspid valve infective endocarditis should raise suspicion for the presence of a patent foramen ovale, a multisite infective endocarditis, a contiguous spread of infection or an endocarditis complicated by perforation. A proper clinical evaluation should also include an assessment of the criteria for sepsis. Concomitant sepsis and the patient's hemodynamic tolerance will affect timing of surgery. The clinician should look for pathophysiological changes associated with infective endocarditis, such as those enumerated in the modified Duke Criteria [17], but also for indicators of prognosis. Examples of combined diagnostic and prognostic findings include right-heart failure caused by tricuspid insufficiency, hepatocellular dysfunction, splenomegaly and cachexia. Another essential role of careful physical examination is to identify or confirm a source of infection or portal of entry. Up to 90% of infective endocarditis cases are caused by the bacteria staphylococci and streptococci, which typically enter the bloodstream from the skin or mucosal surfaces [18, 19]. In 35 to 60% of cases, a portal of entry cannot be ascertained [18, 19]. In patients with known substance use disorder, a wide spectrum of cutaneous manifestations of parental drug abuse may be observed at injection sites. Examples include skin popping (subcutaneous injection), muscle popping (intramuscular injection), ulcers, hyperpigmentation or track marks on the arms, legs, neck, genitalia, inguinal area or between the fingers and toes [20].

3.2 Laboratory testing

The routine preoperative laboratory testing ordered for patients undergoing cardiac surgery should be performed. This includes complete blood count, platelet count, identification of blood group, coagulation panel, as well as a comprehensive metabolic panel. In the context of infective endocarditis, a baseline procalcitonin and C-reactive protein levels should be obtained. These two inflammatory markers can have an influence on decisions regarding management. In the preoperative period, they have a prognostic value correlating with disease severity and can provide another argument for optimal surgical timing. In the postoperative period, they have a prognostic value correlating with resolution of illness and can therefore help monitor treatment response, either hinting towards a recovery or recurrent infection and treatment failure [21–23].

Serum albumin is closely linked to the patient's metabolic status. Hypoalbuminemia can indicate a hepatic insult, an immune disorder or a sepsis-induced catabolism [24]. Low serum albumin levels can also affect pharmacokinetics and pharmacodynamics by decreasing the extent of antibiotic bound to albumin, which increases the unbound fraction of the drug. Unlike the bound fraction of the drug, the unbound fraction is the only fraction available for distribution and clearance from the plasma. Low serum albumin is likely to increase the total volume of distribution and clearance of an antibiotic, which would translate to lower antibacterial exposures that might compromise the efficacy of the treatment [25].

Preoperative liver function tests are essential when planning for surgery of right-sided endocarditis, mainly for two reasons: (i) Right-sided endocarditis in non-drug addict patients without significant medical history is very uncommon; the average patient affected by tricuspid valve endocarditis often has a debilitated medical condition: immune disorder, substance use disorder (drugs and alcohol), cirrhosis, hemodialysis, poor nutritional status and cachexia. (ii) Tricuspid valve endocarditis can, if associated with significant tricuspid insufficiency or right-heart failure, alter hepatic function secondary to hepatic venous congestion. A liver panel should still be performed even in the absence of ascites or jaundice to rule out a subclinical liver insult: thrombopenia, abnormal increase in international normalized ratio (INR), hypoalbuminemia, hepatic cytolysis, pancreatic enzymatic reaction and decrease in factor V. Such findings should warn of an increased risk to develop an acute liver failure or significant coagulopathy during or after the surgery.

3.3 Toxicology screening

In cases where illicit drug use is still suspected (but denied by the patient), a urine drug screen can be done. It will detect evidence of recent cocaine, cannabis, opioids, barbiturates and benzodiazepines use. Detecting and assessing illicit drug use is very important to ensure a proper and individualized therapeutic approach. The perioperative management of patients suffering from drug addiction is fundamentally different from that of non-drug addict patients, both from a medical and surgical perspective. This will be discussed in detail in a subsequent section.

3.4 Microbiology

A systemic infection workup should be performed in order to obtain a complete microbial profile: nasal and rectal swabs, cytobacteriological examination of urine

(CBEU), cytobacteriological examination of the sputum (CBES), blood cultures and serology testing. As a general rule, two sets of blood cultures should be collected immediately and a third one at least 1 hour apart. These blood cultures should be obtained within the first 24 hours of hospital admission. It is well recognized that the sensitivity of blood cultures is largely related to antibiotic uptake prior to blood collection, but also to the volume of the blood sample: 10 mL per blood culture bottle is needed for optimal diagnostic sensitivity [26].

Approximately 5% of case of suspected infective endocarditis yield negative blood culture results, which is often due to prior antibiotic therapy [27]. This should prompt an extension in the duration of incubation of blood culture bottles and ordering a list of molecular tests for culture-negative endocarditis [27]. Two molecular techniques can be used: polymerase chain reaction (PCR), which can either be broad-range or pathogen-specific, and serologic assays, which are especially useful in the presence of intracellular organisms such as Coxiella or Bartonella spp. [28].

While the most common etiologic organism of tricuspid valve endocarditis is Staphylococcus aureus (**Table 1**), polymicrobial infections are also frequent [29]. Fungal endocarditis is a rare but life-threatening condition with a poor prognosis and a mortality rate up to 54% [30]. It should be suspected in the following clinical scenarios: illicit drug use, immunosuppression and/or neutropenia, malignant hemopathies or long-term central venous catheter use. In these cases, serology tests

Organism	Incidence	Risk factors	Other features
Staphylococcus aureus	40–45%	Skin lesion, IVDU (especially MRSA), indwelling prosthetic device (vascular catheters, intracardiac devices, orthopedic prostheses)	Most prevalent pathogen
Coagulase-negative Staphylococcus	5%	Alcoholism, prosthetic valves, indwelling vascular catheters	
Streptococci (especially *Streptococcus pneumoniae*)	30–35%	Alcoholism, prosthetic valves, indwelling vascular catheters, poor dentition	More dominant in left-sided IE
Pseudomonas aeruginosa and other gram-negative bacteria	10%	Neutropenia or other immunodeficiency, advanced age, pancreatobiliary tract disease, severe burns, indwelling central venous or urinary catheter, traumatic wounds that have been contaminated with fresh water	Commonly hospital-acquired (especially in ICU)
Fungi	1–10%	Indwelling central venous catheters, IVDU, prosthetic heart valves or other valvular disease, cancer chemotherapy	Relatively high mortality, incidence rising due to immunocompromised, aging population and intracardiac devices

ICU: intensive care unit; IE: infective endocarditis; IVDU: intravenous drug use; MRSA: methicillin-resistant S. aureus. *Adapted from "Preeminence of S. aureus in infective endocarditis: a 1-year population-based survey," by C. Selton-Suty et al., 2012, Clin Infect Dis., 54(9):1230–9. and from "Trends in Infective Endocarditis in California and New York State" by N. Toyoda et al., 2017, JAMA, 25;317(16):1652–1660. CC BY-NC.*

Table 1.
Common causative microorganisms for right-sided infective endocarditis.

for Aspergillus and Candida spp. should be obtained, in addition to the serum galactomannan antigen test (Aspergillus spp). In case of a negative preliminary workup for fungal infections, β-d-Glucan is an attractive antigen found in cell walls of a broad range of fungal agents and can then be considered [31].

Serological testing for human immunodeficiency virus (HIV)-1 and HIV-2 should be obtained, especially in patients with drug use disorders. Preoperative testing not only helps with patients' management, but it also raises awareness among healthcare providers and prepares them to readily apply the principles of postexposure management in the event of occupational exposure to blood.

3.5 Imaging investigations

3.5.1 Echocardiographic imaging

Transthoracic echocardiogram is the diagnostic procedure of choice and is often sufficient to assess and characterize the pathologic lesions [32, 33]. This is especially true in patients with tricuspid valve endocarditis since this patient population is typically young, has a lower body habitus and larger vegetations [34]. Despite the good performance of transthoracic echocardiogram, transoesophageal echocardiogram has a higher sensitivity −90% compared to 50% for transthoracic echocardiogram- and is better for detecting certain diagnosing features of endocarditis [34]. It is particularly useful for: (i) recognizing subaortic complications, abscesses or fistulas, (ii) ruling out pulmonary valve endocarditis and (iii) better visualizing pacemaker leads and prosthetic valves [35]. It is essential to obtain a detailed anatomical assessment of all the cardiac valves and surrounding structures prior to surgery in order to avoid finding unexpected tissue damage during surgical exploration and avoid unplanned surgical steps. For that reason, transoesophageal echocardiogram should be seen as complimentary to transthoracic echocardiogram [36, 37].

3.5.2 Other imaging workup

In theory, cerebral imaging has little value in right-sided infective endocarditis but it should be done in the presence of any focal neurologic deficit. Cerebral lesions, depending on their extent and severity, may affect timing of surgery or may even be a contraindication to surgery. In addition, any sign of brain involvement in right-sided infective endocarditis suggests a concomitant left-sided endocarditis or the spread of the infection from a right-sided valve to left-sided structures.

With tricuspid valve endocarditis, a computer tomography scan of the chest, abdomen and pelvis must be obtained to evaluate for septic emboli, infarcts or abscesses (**Table 2**).

^{18}F-fluorodeoxyglucose positron emission tomography-computed tomography (FDG PET-CT) has been included into the recommended workup for patients with suspected infective endocarditis, according to major society guidelines [38, 39]. In the context of inflammation or infection, ^{18}F-fluorodeoxyglucose, an analogue of glucose, is primarily taken up by activated neutrophils which exhibit enhanced glycolysis, hence acting as a radiotracer. There are two main indications for performing an FDG PET-CT: (i) to supplement the echocardiogram in characterizing intracardiac infections, especially in the endocardium, and (ii) to detect clinically silent disseminated disease [40]. However, ambiguity remains regarding the optimal use and timing of this imaging modality [38, 39]. In addition, FDG PET-CT is non-contributory for

Valvular/Local	Nonvalvular/Peripheral
Tricuspid insufficiency Tricuspid stenosis Valve destruction Leaflet perforation Periannular abscess formation	Pulmonary: embolism, infiltrates, exudates, abscess, cavitation, aneurysms, pleural effusion. Systemic embolism and infarcts (most often paradoxical embolus via patent foramen ovale or intracardiac shunt) High degree atrioventricular block Septic shock Multiorgan failure

Table 2.
Major complications of tricuspid valve infective endocarditis.

cerebral imaging in this setting given the principles of brain metabolism. Its usefulness is also very limited in the early postoperative period owing to the acute sterile inflammatory changes induced by surgical insults, which increase the likelihood of a false-positive finding [41].

The addition of radiolabeled white blood cell scintigraphy looks promising, especially for differentiating between active infection and inflammation. However, its complexity, limited availability and lack of adaptation are the main challenges to its use [42].

3.6 Intraoperative investigations

In cases in which definitive microbiologic diagnosis cannot be established preoperatively based on culture or serology alone, tissue samples must be collected intraoperatively from the infected valve/tissues or vegetations. These specimens should be sent fresh in appropriate sterile containers for both histopathological and microbiological examinations, but the largest sample should be sent to the molecular diagnostic unit to perform a broad-range PCR. This highly sensitive technique amplifies small quantities of 16SrDNA (for bacteria) or 18SrDNA (for fungi), which can then be sequenced for specific pathogen identification [43].

Achieving quality verbal and written communication between the pathologist, biologist and surgeon is crucial to avoid any loss of information, diagnostic error, and patient harm. Multiple components should be clarified, including pertinent clinical information, intraoperative observations, precise location of tissue removal, diagnostic uncertainty, specific tests that are required, expectation of report turnaround time, etc. [44, 45]. The pathologist and biologist should understand the role of the requested laboratory tests in the diagnostic process and therapeutic strategy, and their importance for antibiotic stewardship.

3.7 Postoperative investigations

Treatment response must be assessed postoperatively with serial complete blood counts, procalcitonin and C-reactive protein levels. After hospital discharge, both clinical and echocardiographic follow-up are recommended to monitor potential complications, such as recurrence of infection, persistent valve dysfunction, heart failure, development of new vegetations, etc. International guidelines recommend obtaining a baseline transthoracic echocardiogram at the completion of antimicrobial therapy, followed by serial examinations at 1, 3, 6 and 12 months [46]. In the presence of prosthetic valve or other biomaterial, a PET scan can be obtained 3 months after surgery to rule out a recurrent infection with higher sensitivity. However, it should be interpreted carefully by an experienced user and images should be compared to any previously obtained sequence to avoid any false-positive result caused by normal postsurgical aseptic inflammatory changes [41].

4. Guidelines on the surgical management of tricuspid valve endocarditis in adults

4.1 Indications

Any decision about surgical intervention should be made by a heart valve multidisciplinary team. Decisions on surgical intervention are complex and depend on many clinical and prognostic factors that vary among patients, including causative organism, vegetation size, presence of perivalvular infection, presence of embolism or heart failure, age, noncardiac comorbidities, and available surgical expertise. Decisions on the indication and timing of surgical intervention should be determined by a multispecialty team with expertise in cardiology, imaging, cardiothoracic surgery, and infectious diseases. Indications for surgical intervention in right-sided infective endocarditis include the following [39, 47]:

- Presence of highly resistant organisms;
- Persistent bacteremia for >5–7 days despite adequate antimicrobial therapy;
- Right heart failure due to severe tricuspid regurgitation with poor response to medical therapy;
- Paravalvular abscess or destructive penetrating lesions;
- Heart block;
- Recurrent septic pulmonary emboli;
- Large, persistent vegetations (>20 mm).

The first five clinical scenarios are a Class I indication for early surgery according to the 2020 American College of Cardiology/American Heart Association guidelines for the management of valvular heart disease [48]. Early valve surgery represents a surgery that is done during the initial hospital course, prior to completion of antimicrobial therapy. Reasons to consider early surgery are to avoid progressive heart failure and irreversible structural damage caused by the infection. Early surgery for recurrent pulmonary emboli is a class 2a indication according to those same guidelines, while early surgery for large (>20 mm) vegetations is a class 2b indication. In patients with implanted electronic devices, infection of the entire system is likely and this mandates complete removal of leads and generator in order to eradicate the infection (Class I). Because of its high success rate and low complication rate, interventional transvenous extraction of pacemaker leads is favored over surgical extraction.

The 2015 European Society of Cardiology guidelines for the management of infective endocarditis list three Class IIa indications for surgical intervention of right-sided infective endocarditis [38]:

- Right heart failure due to severe tricuspid regurgitation with poor response to medical therapy;
- Presence of highly resistant organisms that are difficult to eradicate;
- Persistent bacteraemia >7 days despite adequate antimicrobial therapy;
- Tricuspid valve vegetations >20 mm that persist after recurrent pulmonary emboli.

4.2 Contraindications

In theory, there are very few contraindications to surgical intervention for endocarditis. However, in practice, some clinical scenarios present difficult dilemmas. Patients >65 years of age have an increased risk of infective endocarditis and their overall outcome is less favorable due to the presence of comorbidities, delayed presentation and frequent history of antimicrobial use. However, age per se is not a preclusion to surgical intervention [49]. Risk stratification models such as the Society of Thoracic Surgeons Endocarditis Score are available to predict morbidity and mortality risks and to assist in patient-centered decision-making.

Recurrent endocarditis due to continued drug abuse is not an absolute contraindication to surgery, but many surgeons may see this intervention as futile. The ESC guidelines recommend avoiding surgical intervention in patients who continue to inject drugs, except in the situations mentioned previously that prompt early intervention [38]. As part of decision-making about reoperation, the ACC/AHA guidelines include a Class I recommendation to consult with experts in addiction medicine about the patient's long-term ability to refrain from drug use before deciding on surgical candidacy. Cardiac surgery is contraindicated for at least one month after intracranial hemorrhage unless neurosurgical or endovascular intervention can be performed to reduce bleeding risk [48]. After an ischaemic stroke, surgery is only contraindicated if there is extensive neurological damage and if the neurological prognosis is judged too poor.

5. General principles of surgical management

Those principles follow the basic rules of the surgical management of contaminated and infected operative fields.

1. Whenever possible and if permitted by hemodynamic status, surgery should be delayed until bacterial shedding is decreased. This is usually achieved within a couple days of effective antibiotic therapy. That being said, a surgical delay that is justified by the vain hope of achieving a sterile operative field and that results in cardiac tissue destruction and deterioration in the overall clinical condition may cause significant harm to the patient.

2. Be aware that preoperative imaging always underestimates the severity of the lesions. In other words, one should expect to find more tissue damage and destruction.

3. "It's like going to war.": surgery for infective endocarditis has a higher burden of unexpected findings and complications compared to other types of cardiac procedures.

4. Regarding cannulation strategy for cardiopulmonary bypass, a bicaval cannulation is a safer choice owing to its versatility.

5. Regarding cardioplegia, cases should be considered individually since multiple strategies are possible. The chosen approach should however be shaped around the surgeon comfort level and should allow to safely perform a complex surgery.

6. Retrograde cardioplegia may wash out distal emboli from the coronary ostia and is therefore an attractive option in combined aortotricuspid valve endocarditis.

7. Minimal manipulation of cardiac structures until cardioplegic arrest to avoid embolism.

8. Complete extraction of prosthetic material and debridement of all infected and necrotic tissue.

9. Generous irrigation of the operative field with antibiotic solution and scrubbing of healthy tissue with antibiotic-soaked gauze.

10. A non-antibacterial lavage with non-antibacterial solutions (povidone iodine, superoxidised water, etc.) may also be used but has been shown to be less effective at reducing surgical site infection compared to antibacterial solutions [50].

11. Thorough intraoperative histology and microbiology testing; this must be done even if a causative agent was identified preoperatively in order to rule out a polymicrobial infection or the presence of fastidious microorganisms that did not grow on initial blood cultures. The results of these microbiology tests will influence duration of therapy. Guidelines suggest that if resected valve tissue is culture positive or if a perivalvular abscess is found, then an entire course of antimicrobial therapy is reasonable after surgery [39]. All appropriate containers as well as specimen collection and transportation supplies should be available to avoid wasting samples. These should also be clearly labeled.

12. The surgical instruments that are used for the first part of the surgery- until the debridement of infected tissue- should be replaced for the second half of the procedure to avoid contaminating the operative field.

13. For tricuspid valve repair strategies:

    - Avoid the use of braided sutures as they are more prone to bacterial adherence [51];

- Favor the use of interrupted sutures [52, 53];
- Use pericardium strips or pledgets to consolidate suture lines.

14. Providing an adequate nutritional support is crucial owing to the hypermetabolic state seen in sepsis [54, 55].

15. Insertion of a peripherally inserted central catheter (PICC) line or port-a-cath should be seriously considered and discussed among the multidisciplinary team for postoperative continuation of antibiotic therapy.

16. The risk of reinfection or recurrent infective endocarditis is a major concern; however, this risk decreases over time [56].

5.1 Characteristics of tricuspid valve infective endocarditis

5.1.1 Surgical approach

In the majority of cases, a midline sternotomy is performed. However, a minimally invasive surgical approach has been described for isolated tricuspid valve intervention [57]. Through our experience, we find that both techniques can be safely and effectively performed, but each has its own advantages and disadvantages. Ultimately, the choice of approach should take into consideration the surgeon's comfort level, patient's characteristics and patient's preference. Minimally invasive surgery is an excellent option for both redo and primary surgery cases. However, as stated previously, tissue damage and destruction if often found to be more severe than expected; the operative field should therefore be accessible enough to perform a complete debridement and repair.

5.1.2 Cardiopulmonary bypass

- Bicaval cannulation provides an unobstructed surgical field. These cannulas typically have a right-angled tip to facilitate exposure.
- Vacuum-assisted veinous drainage will facilitate venous drainage, especially for the subdiaphragmatic venous circulation which can be subjected to congestion secondary to the retrograde flow from tricuspid regurgitation [58]. Adequate cardiac decompression can even be achieved without snaring the vena cava [59].
- Vasoplegic syndrome following cardiopulmonary bypass remains a serious and relatively frequent occurrence that will further complicate postoperative hemodynamic management. Adding hemofiltration, leukocyte-depleting filters and/or cytokine filters (CytoSorb®) to the pump circuit is particularly appealing in this patient population because of their pro-inflammatory state and hypervolemic status. However, evidence to support their use is still lacking [60, 61].

5.1.3 Cardioplegia

Aortic cross-clamping and cardioplegic arrest are not required in isolated tricuspid valve disease; the procedure can therefore be done off-pump. This has several advantages:

- It avoids triggering a second "inflammatory hit" that would otherwise exacerbate the hyperinflammatory state and vasoplegia caused by the bacteremia;
- It avoids inducing myocardial ischemia associated with the use of cardiopulmonary bypass;
- It allows real-time monitoring of the cardiac rhythm, thus allows to troubleshoot rhythm disturbances when suturing around the triangle of Koch.

If a more complex surgery is needed (e.g. homograft replacement), aortic cross-clamping becomes necessary; it will allow the surgeon to work on an immobile field, thus enhance precision of hand gestures. If the infection affects other valves, the tricuspid valve should be the last one to address, and if possible, after unclamping. Aortic cross-clamping and cardioplegic arrest are also required when a patent foramen ovale is diagnosed on echocardiogram in order to prevent venous air embolism or embolic debris from the vegetations to paradoxically enter the systemic circulation. If there is uncertainty regarding the extent of tissue lesions, a safe approach would be to perform the surgery while on-pump, still with bicaval cannulation, which will allow for any valvular correction. The choice of cardioplegia should be at the discretion of the surgical team.

5.1.4 Incision and exposure

The right atriotomy is performed in parallel to the atrioventricular groove, at least 1 cm away from it in order to avoid injury to the right coronary artery during closure. In case of a redo operation, the atrioventricular groove is often difficult to visualize because of adhesions. The atriotomy can then be caried out along the virtual line that connects the two venous cannulas. A proper exposure will help achieve a thorough inspection of the cardiac structures and tissues. It includes a functional assessment of the tricuspid valve, which can be achieved using hand-held retractors, a valve retractor system such as the Cosgrove retractor, or multiple suspension sutures. This step is crucial as it will determine the optimal surgical approach (repair or replacement) to address the valvular pathology.

5.1.5 Surgical closure

Most often, a single continuous prolene suture is enough to close the right atriotomy. However, the free edges of the atriotomy might appear very thin with right atrial enlargement, in which case a double running suture might be necessary, with or without surgical adhesive.

6. Surgical management of tricuspid valve infective endocarditis

Two scenarios can be encountered when determining optimal surgical treatment for tricuspid valve endocarditis:

1. If the endocarditis is considered sterile: The main concerns at that point are potential hemodynamic instabilities and the risk of embolism. The purpose of surgery is therefore to correct the tricuspid valve pathology but it will typically

not be performed in emergent situations. Surgical timing remains a key element to optimize outcomes: surgery must be offered early, whenever indications are met, but before patients develop right heart failure. The choice of surgical technique should take into consideration the degree of tissue damage, the patient's clinical status, their age, their burden of comorbidities and their risk of recurrence.

2. If the endocarditis is not considered sterile: The main objective is to debride all devitalized and infected tissue, such as vegetations or abscesses. Tissue that appears edematous or abnormal should also be debrided. In addition to correcting the tricuspid valve pathology, the goal of surgery is to also avoid implanting any prosthetic material into an infected area.

6.1 Therapeutic options

6.1.1 Tricuspid valvulectomy

Proposed by Arbulu and colleagues [62], this surgical technique is rarely performed today. The goal is to excise the tricuspid valve without replacing it. It was performed mostly in patients with intractable endocarditis and ongoing drug abuse who had a high risk of relapse or recurrent infection. Results were better than expected and the reported mortality –29% on the first case series- was mainly due to non-cardiac complications. The team of surgeons who pioneered this operation still defend its merits, but its adoption has been largely decreased with the advent of tricuspid valve repair techniques that do not involve the use of prosthetic material [63]. The rapid advances in transcatheter heart valve interventions might give tricuspid valvulectomy a second chance in cases of severe and complex tricuspid valve infective endocarditis: in a double-stage procedure, a tricuspid valvulectomy, performed first, would allow for an effective control of the infection, followed by a transcatheter valve intervention to address the tricuspid regurgitation.

6.1.2 Tricuspid valve repair

Tricuspid valve repair can be achieved using different techniques:

6.1.2.1 Vegetectomy/suture/patch

Vegetations are often found on the valve leaflets. Resection of the vegetation at its base can lead to a leaflet defect (depending on the level of leaflet involvement). A small defect can be sutured directly [64, 65]. As long as there is no chordal resection, larger defects may require pericardial patching (e.g. glutaraldehyde-treated autologous pericardium) in order to avoid leaflet distortion. Patching can be done using either interrupted or continuous sutures [66]. In case of annular erosion or abscess, all infected tissue should be debrided until a healthy circumference of tissue is visualized. The remaining defect should be patched, and the annulus, reconstructed: the preserved tricuspid leaflet can then be reattached to the neo-annulus.

6.1.2.2 Chordal damage

Rupture of chordae tendineae is rare and is usually associated with a free edge destruction of the leaflet. This can be addressed with a leaflet reconstruction using a patch and Gore-Tex chordoplasty. Artificial chords made of polytetrafluoroethylene (PTFE) have good long-term durability and are relatively resistant to infection [67].

6.1.2.3 Annuloplasty

In the setting of annular abnormality (i.e. dilation or distortion), an attempt should be made to restore annular rigidity, both for short-term and long-term benefits. The following techniques can be used: (i) commissural plication or (ii) DeVega annuloplasty. For commissural plication, an X suture is placed at the level of the postero-septal and/or anteroposterior commissure. The depth of the suture determines the degree of annular size reduction. The DeVega annuloplasty consists of running two parallel sutures between the postero-septal commissure to the antero-septal commissure. The two sutures should run in opposite directions, the first suture starting on the postero-septal commissure and the second, on the antero-septal commissure. The sutures are then tied using pledget reinforcement, while using an angled Hegar dilator or a ring sizer (32 mm for men and 28 mm for women) to help accurately size the annulus. Synthetic pledgets can be replaced with pericardial pledgets to further reduce the risk of reinfection [68].

6.1.2.4 Annuloplasty ring

The decision to implant a prosthetic ring should be considered with caution and weighed against the risk of reinfection.

6.1.2.5 Suture bicuspidization

The Kay technique is one way to achieve bicuspidization. It involves an annulorrhaphy of the posterior segment which results in obliterating the posterior leaflet. The Alfieri stitch, originately described for the mitral valve, can also be used for the tricuspid valve, with satistifying results [69, 70]. It consists in suturing together the middle point of the free edges of the tricuspid leaflets in order to create a coaptation zone in the center. This also results in 2 or 3 tricuspid orifices, giving the valve a clover shape. Indeed, this technique is sometimes referred to as "the Clover Technique. Bicuspidization of the tricuspid valve seems to be well tolerated by patients [71]. These techniques and their principles are being applied to the field of transcatheter intervention [72].

6.1.2.6 Tricuspid valve replacement

The key point is to avoid injury to the conduction system. In order to achieve that, two suturing techniques have been described: (i) placing the stitches into the fibrous tissue along the septal leaflet or (ii) implanting the prosthetic valve above the level of the coronary sinus, leaving the latter on the ventricular side.

6.2 Selection of a substitute

6.2.1 Mitral homograft replacement

A tricuspid homograft is difficult to preserve because the leaflets are very thin and the chordae tendinae, too numerous. The surgical technique is also challenging, making it a suboptimal option in emergent situations. On the opposite, tricuspid valve replacement with mitral valve homograft is feasible [73, 74]. The chords can be implanted before fixing the homograft to the tricuspid annulus, or vice versa [73]. The homograft can either be placed in the anatomical or the anti-anatomical position; the optimal orientation being controversial, the choice remains at the surgeon's discretion. However, the benefits of adding an annuloplasty ring are well established [75]. A main disadvantage of this substitute is that it's not widely available in the required sizes for the tricuspid annulus.

6.2.2 Inverted aortic valve xenograft

Implantation of a stentless aortic root prothesis using an inversion technique has been described as an alternative to mitral homograft replacement [76]. The sinuses of Valsalva should be trimmed prior to implantation, leaving only the commissural posts suspending the aortic valve within. These posts will serve as chordal attachments. The xenograft is positioned, sutured in place and the commissures are attached to the right ventricular cavity.

6.2.3 Mechanical prosthesis

The main challenge is the requirement for lifelong oral anticoagulation using a vitamin K antagonist. This is a serious concern, especially in the tricuspid position because the tricuspid valve is a low flow valve, which increases the risk of thromboembolic events. During implantation, particular care must be taken to ensure normal leaflet excursion.

6.2.4 Bioprosthesis

These do not require lifelong anticoagulation; however, vitamin K antagonists should be considered in all patients for 3 to 6 months after surgery. Other advantages include:

i. A good long-term durability in the tricuspid position given the low flows;

ii. An excellent anchoring frame for future transcatheter valve therapy;

iii. In case of a recurrent endocarditis, the infection will tend affect the leaflets rather than the annulus.

During implantation, the struts of the bioprosthesis should be positioned so they straddle the conduction tissue, which helps to avoid heart block.

6.3 Transcatheter valve therapy

Many cases of infective endocarditis post-transcatheter heart valve interventions have been described, but literature specifically describing the use of transcatheter valve therapy to address endocarditis remains scarce. The reason probably stems from the fact that infective endocarditis often involves tissue damage which requires surgical debridement. In addition, transcatheter tricuspid valve therapy is still in its early stages of development [77]. Current tricuspid valve catheter devices can be divided into four categories, according to their mode of action: annuloplasty devices, edge-to-edge repair devices, coaptation devices and caval valve devices. These devices can address the tricuspid regurgitation, but not the tissue lesions, thus representing an incomplete therapeutic solution to a complex condition. Recently, a percutaneous vacuum-assisted device coupled with a veno-venous extracorporeal system (AngioVac, AngioDynamics) was introduced for the removal of right-sided intracardiac masses. The system is inserted through the femoral vein and consists of a 22 French coil-reinforced drainage canula. Several case series showed a high success rate for debulking large vegetations (2 cm on average), leaving small residual vegetations which can be treated with antibiotics [47, 77]. This promising therapeutic avenue could certainly benefit patients who have a prohibitive surgical risk and those in whom implantation of prosthetic material is to be avoided (e.g. ongoing drug abuse). Furthermore, percutaneous aspiration of vegetations may help reduce the immediate risk of septic embolization while allowing surgeons to postpone definitive intervention at a later date, once the clinical status is improved. In cases where there is no need for surgical debridement, this definitive intervention could even be a transcatheter heart valve intervention. However, percutaneous vacuum-assisted devices have their own potential adverse effects, including vascular access complications or disruption of the vegetation leading to pulmonary embolization [47, 77]. Larger prospective studies are needed to determine their safety and efficacy.

6.4 Outcomes

The clinical outcomes of surgical interventions on the tricuspid valve are difficult to interpret. This is in part explained by the fact that most published data come from small case series, while larger studies often do not exclude combined mitral and tricuspid cases [78–81]. Operative mortality for tricuspid valve infective endocarditis ranges between 6% and 30% but is rarely precipitated by the tricuspid intervention itself. The most common risk factors for operative mortality include multivalvular endocarditis and preoperative multiorgan failure. The postoperative and middle-term prognosis are influenced by right ventricular function and the presence of pulmonary arterial hypertension.

7. Specific management considerations

7.1 Intravenous drug users

Drug use disorder is the persistent and compulsive use of drugs despite substantial harm and adverse consequences as a result of their use. Patients suffering from this disorder become dependent on the intense but short-lived feelings of pleasure derived from surges of activation of the brain's reward system. Despite the knowledge of certain risk factors, there is not a definitive socio-professional or psychological profile that perfectly predicts drug addiction. Drug addiction can affect anyone. However, it is rarely openly disclosed by patients, and is instead presented as being occasional/recreational. People with substance dependency often report feelings of guilt and shame. There are many barriers to getting help, including discrimination, misunderstanding or fear of possible criminal consequences. Patients with drug addiction who are diagnosed with infective endocarditis often present at an advanced stage that requires emergent management. This context is not suitable for an abrupt drug discontinuation. A proper drug weaning and tapering should be consensual and carefully planned. It is a long and difficult process that should not be disrupted by a concomitant disease.

The provider-patient interaction in the presence of drug addiction can be defined on three levels: (a) relational, (b) medical and (c) social.

7.1.1 Relational considerations

The context is certainly delicate. Unconscious bias may lead to poorer interactions. Concomitant psychological or psychiatric disorders may be precipitated into a crisis state or an acute phase of symptoms during hospital admission. Health care providers will have to face many interpersonal challenges: establishing trust and showing compassion while setting strict relational boundaries and therapeutic principles. It is a competent adult's prerogative to give, refuse or withdraw consent to health care, and this must be a voluntary decision free of any coercion or pressure. Ethical uncertainty can arise for health care providers when patients decline treatments that appear to be in their best interests, however, there is a strong obligation to honor the patient's wishes. In order to avoid any ethical conflicts and to prevent patient harm, continued and open discussions with the patient must occur along every step of the therapeutic process to demonstrate mutual respect and even out power imbalances.

Health care providers should also be appropriately trained in withdrawal management, including recognizing the physical and psychological symptoms of withdrawal, applying behavioral management strategies and using the right medications for alleviating common withdrawal symptoms. Drug withdrawal can occur at any stage of the hospital stay, including postoperatively. In order to maximize patient and worker safety, patients with drug abuse disorder should be enrolled in an inpatient withdrawal management program. These services are staffed by an experienced and dedicated multidisciplinary team that may include nurses, nurse practitioners, physicians, social workers, recreational therapists, counselors and spiritual care professionals. In terms of logistics, visitors on the unit should be closely monitored as they may smuggle drugs to patients. Patients may also leave the unit to obtain substances outside on hospital property. Having institutional policies about visitors and patients' entries and exits might facilitate collaboration with staff, as well as optimize effective prevention of relapse during inpatient therapy.

7.1.2 Medical considerations

7.1.2.1 Serology

Obtaining serology testing is crucial, not only to help with patients' management (morbidity status, immunodeficiency versus immunocompetence), but to also protect healthcare providers in the event of occupational exposure to blood.

7.1.2.2 Surgery

Tricuspid valve repair techniques should be the preferred approach in this patient population despite the presence of a fastidious organism, because the risks of a recurrent infection are very high. The implantation of prosthetic material should be seen as a last resort.

7.1.2.3 Prescription drug interactions

Identification of potential drug interactions must be part of the preoperative evaluation. It is very important to gather a detailed and complete drug history (name, type, frequency), including of illicit drugs, over-the-counter and herbal products. Opiate addicts may have a skewed perception of pain and may have developed resistance to analgesic therapy [82]. The latter can easily become a source of tension, or even conflict, between the patient and primary care team: on one hand, the patient may be convinced that staff is intentionally letting them suffer (paranoid thinking), while on the other hand, the staff believe that the patient is exhibiting an exaggerated pain behavior in order to obtain more opioid analgesics. In addition, providers are often caught between a rock and a hard place: dosages should be high enough to prevent withdrawal while avoiding an overdose.

7.1.2.4 Venous access

Obtaining venous access is often difficult owing to the chronic damage to the peripheral venous system from intravenous drug use and frequent sites of vein thrombosis. A peripherally inserted central catheter (PICC) line or an implanted port (also called a "port" or "port-a-cath") placement could therefore be necessary for the completion of long-term antibiotic therapy. Paradoxically, these indwelling catheters provide a tempting access for continued drug abuse and are therefore a significant risk factor for recurrent infection in patients who decide to misuse them.

7.2 Social considerations

The follow-up of intravenous drug abusers after hospital discharge should include: wound care, antibiotic treatment, psychological support and drug rehabilitation. Without this follow-up, management remains incomplete and will most likely fail. Indeed, prognosis of drug addicts following hospital discharge worsens over time because they are in a more vulnerable state: the accumulated desire to abuse will be maximal. This increased risk of relapse following hospital discharge should be openly discussed with the patient as soon as possible, even as early as hospital admission.

7.3 Cardiac implantable electronic devices

7.3.1 Epidemiology and diagnosis

The reported prevalence of cardiac device-related infective endocarditis is between 0.5% and 7% [83]. This phenomenon is on the rise despite strict sterile surgical techniques and infection prevention and control practices such as systematic antibiotic prophylaxis. The increased incidence of cardiac device-related infective endocarditis is certainly linked to an aging population with multiple chronic conditions and increased metabolic and functional vulnerability [83]. Other patient-related risk factors include female gender, diabetes mellitus, heart failure, active cancer and long-term glucocorticoid therapy [84]. Procedure-related risk factors include fever at the time of device implantation, prior temporary internal pacing, implantation of more than two electrodes and hematoma formation at the pocket region [84, 85]. The risk of infection is multiplied by two after a generator replacement or a surgical reexploration [84, 85]. Admission mortality rates associated with cardiac device-related infective endocarditis have been reported to be between 3% and 8% [86]. The financial costs associated with this condition are also significant (length of hospital stay, investigations, long-term antibiotic treatment, surgery, etc.) and reflect the potential severity of the infection burden [87].

The most common causative agents are coagulase-negative staphylococci (40–60%), S. aureus (20–30%), gram-negative bacilli such as Klebsiella pneumoniae, Pseudomonas aeruginosa or Proteus mirabilis (10%), and more rarely, polymicrobial. In 30% of cases, there is no identifiable organism, which is typically seen when empiric antibiotics are started before collecting blood cultures (38). Many recent studies have highlighted the added value of fluorine-18-fluorodeoxyglucose (18F-FDG) positron-emission tomography (PET)/computed tomography (CT) for clinically suspected cardiac device-related infective endocarditis infection cases with diagnostic uncertainty or equivocal findings, to the point where its use has been endorsed by guidelines [88, 89].

7.3.2 Management

Management should be based on a multidisciplinary strategy, involving anesthesia, electrophysiology, cardiac surgery and microbiology [38]. The primum movens is to apply the general principles of management of any prosthesis infection:

1. Intravenous antibiotic treatment (pre and post extraction);

2. Complete extraction of the prosthesis (generator and leads/electrodes);

3. Microbiology testing during the extraction procedure for antibiotic stewardship. Pocket swabs, lead tips and blood samples should be cultured onto a range of media.

The step-by-step approach of the extraction procedure will be determined by the patient's baseline rhythm, the presence or absence of pacemaker dependency, the presence or absence of vegetations on native valves, and the length of time since insertion. The electrophysiologist will help to decide on other factors such as the pacemaker model, type of leads/electrodes, timing of surgery and the location of the new generator. A complete surgical extraction of the material should be performed in order to achieve eradication of the infection and reduce mortality. However, it remains a relatively high-risk intervention. Operative risks are associated with a risk of septic shock secondary to the dissemination of infection from tissue manipulation, surgical wound infection, major hemorrhage from vascular injury, iatrogenic damage to the tricuspid valve, subclavian vein tear or hemothorax [90]. When it comes to lead extraction, the "age" of the lead matters. With early lead infection, the lead will often be covered in vegetations with little adherence to the tricuspid valve; that scenario can be addressed with complete device extraction, vegetation debulking and epicardial

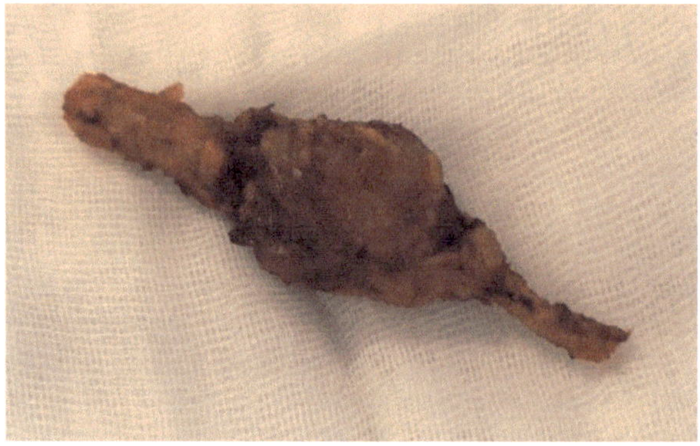

Figure 8.
Infected pacemaker lead with vegetation.

lead placement. On the contrary, an "old" infected lead will often be entrapped to the tricuspid valve by encapsulating fibrous tissue, which significantly complicates the extraction. If the tricuspid valve cannot be safely reconstructed and repaired due to severe adherence, tricuspid valve replacement becomes necessary.

Once the infected leads are removed (**Figure 8**), a decision should be made about replacing them. This will depend on the patient's baseline rhythm and the adopted strategy:

1. No immediate lead reimplantation, as long as the triangle of Koch is left intact. A comprehensive postoperative evaluation should be obtained (electrocardiogram, Holter, electrophysiology study, etc.) to determine if lead reimplantation (endocardial approach or leadless) should be planned at a later stage.

2. Epicardial lead implantation.

3. Endocardial lead and pacemaker reimplantation during the same procedure. The new generator can be placed in the left abdominal wall, behind the insertion of the rectus muscle at the thoracoabdominal junction. Through experience, we found that this anatomical location offers many advantages: it is easily accessible via midline sternotomy, it prevents pacemaker exteriorization and it is generally well tolerated by patients.

Regarding the types of endocardial leads, these can either have a passive fixation or an active fixation (**Figure 9**). Active-fixation leads, also called screw-in leads, are usually preferred. They have extendable screws that can be deployed and fixed on the inside surface of the cardiac chamber. It is worth noting that he stimulation thresholds are usually higher with active-fixation leads compared to passive-fixation leads. If the threshold is too high, the lead should be unscrewed and repositioned. However, the number of attempts is not unlimited; repeated screwing/unscrewing can easily damage the thin wall of the right ventricle. One should also avoid over-torquing to minimize the risk of perforation. This is especially relevant in the context of an infection where tissues are more fragile.

Epicardial leads can also have high stimulation thresholds in the following cases: pericarditis, myocardial inflammation, myocardial edema (prolonged

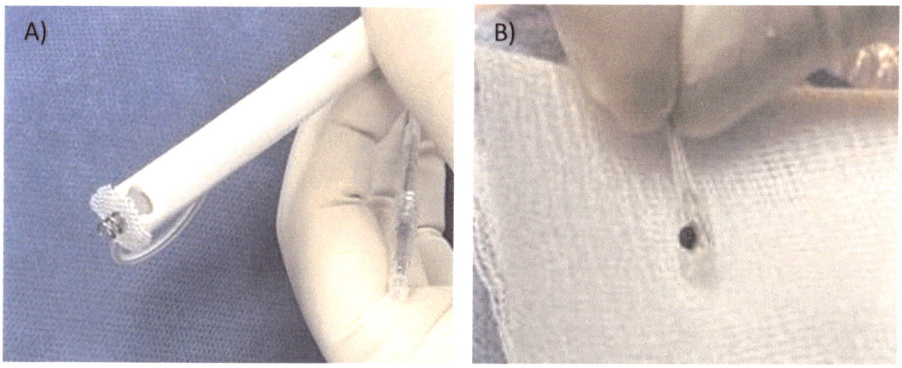

Figure 9.
Active-fixation (A) and passive-fixation (B) pacemaker leads.

cardiopulmonary bypass times or cardioplegia). Repositioning the epicardial leads is challenging in these scenarios given the risk of laceration of the right ventricle; tolerating a sub-optimal threshold is therefore acceptable. Furthermore, adjustments to the pacemaker settings can be made later from the external generator. Having an electrophysiologist or a pacemaker technologist at the time of epicardial lead implantation is therefore not necessary.

Lastly, infection prevention and control measures should be rigorously applied to minimize the risk of recurrence: skin antiseptic preparation, aseptic practices in the operating room, prophylactic antibiotics with coverage against S. aureus and Staphylococcus epidermidis. Local antibiotic usage for infection prophylaxis, in particular pocket irrigation or absorbable antibacterial envelopes, remains controversial but limited reports suggest they may have a benefit, especially in select high-risk patients [91–93].

8. Conclusion

Tricuspid valve infectious endocarditis is an uncommon condition, especially when compared to left-sided endocarditis. However, it is characterized by high morbidity and mortality. The prognosis will be determined by the control of the infection (medical and surgical), surgical timing, appropriate prophylaxis and the risk of recurrence. The therapeutic management is complex and should be provided by a multidisciplinary team, including cardiologists, cardiac surgeons, pathologists, microbiologists and imaging specialists. Patients with a substance use disorder should be referred to addiction services in order to the start the rehabilitation process while in hospital. A close medical and psychosocial follow-up should be offered after hospital discharge. A collaborative multidisciplinary approach is crucial to manage patients with infective endocarditis effectively and was shown to significantly improve their prognosis [94]. This concept, of the so-called "Endocarditis Team", is at the heart of contemporary cardiovascular care and is encountered in other areas, such as transcatheter valve implantations (e.g., the "TAVI Team"). The advent of transcatheter interventions may bring new therapeutic options that will benefit patients who are deemed unfit for surgery.

Author details

Olina Dagher[1,2], Walid Ben Ali[1,3], Nils Perrin[3,4], Nancy Poirier[1,5] and Nicolas Dürrleman[1,3]*

1 Department of Surgery, Montreal Heart Institute, Montreal, Canada

2 Department of Cardiac Sciences, Libin Cardiovascular Institute, Calgary, Canada

3 Structural Heart Program, Montreal Heart Institute, Montreal, Canada

4 Cardiology Division, Geneva University Hospitals, Switzerland

5 Sainte Justine Hospital, Montréal, Canada

*Address all correspondence to: nicodurr@hotmail.com

References

[1] Zubarevich A, Szczechowicz M, Brcic A, et al. Tricuspid valve repair in isolated tricuspid pathology: A 12-year single center experience. Journal of Cardiothoracic Surgery. 2020; **15**(1):330

[2] Tagliari AP, Perez-Camargo D, Taramasso M. Tricuspid regurgitation: When is it time for surgery? Expert Review of Cardiovascular Therapy. 2021; **19**(1):47-59

[3] Chow SCY, Wan S. Commentary: Should prophylactic tricuspid annuloplasty be routinely performed? If so, how? The jury is still out. JTCVS Open. 2021;7:139-140

[4] Mohanan S, Gopalan Nair R, Vellani H, Sanjeev CG, George B, Krishnan MN. Baseline C-reactive protein levels and prognosis in patients with infective endocarditis: A prospective cohort study. Indian Heart Journal. 2018;**70**(Suppl 3):S43-S49

[5] Anwar AM, Geleijnse ML, Soliman OII, et al. Assessment of normal tricuspid valve anatomy in adults by real-time three-dimensional echocardiography. The International Journal of Cardiovascular Imaging. 2007; **23**:717-724

[6] Hahn RT. State-of-the-art review of echocardiographic imaging in the evaluation and treatment of functional tricuspid regurgitation. Circulation. Cardiovascular Imaging. 2016;**9**(12): e005332

[7] Pozzoli A, Zuber M, Reisman M, Maisano F, Taramasso M. Comparative anatomy of mitral and tricuspid valve: What can the Interventionlist learn from the surgeon. Frontiers in Cardiovascular Medicine. 2018;**5**:80

[8] Kirklin JW, Barratt-Boyes BG. Cardiac Surgery. New York: Churchill Livingstone; 1993. pp. 589-608

[9] Villablanca PA, Sukhal S, Maitas O, et al. Aorto-right atrial fistula: Late complication of tricuspid valve infective endocarditis. World Journal of Cardiology. 2014;**6**(10):1122-1126

[10] Liesenborghs L, Meyers S, Vanassche T, Verhamme P. Coagulation: At the heart of infective endocarditis. Journal of Thrombosis and Haemostasis. 2020;**18**(5):995-1008

[11] Morrissy SJ, Atkins BZ, Rogers JH. Iatrogenic right coronary artery stenosis resulting from surgical tricuspid valve replacement: Case report and review of the literature. Catheterization and Cardiovascular Interventions. 2014; **84**(7):1110-1114

[12] Anderson RH, Ho SY, Becker AE. Anatomy of the human atrioventricular junctions revisited. The Anatomical Record. 2000;**260**(1):81-91

[13] Anderson RH, Sanchez-Quintana D, Mori S, Cabrera JA, Back SE. Re-evaluation of the structure of the atrioventricular node and its connections with the atrium. Europace. 2020;**22**(5): 821-830

[14] Bru P, Iacono C, Collet F, et al. Endocardite tricuspidienne avec shunt droite-gauche à l'étage auriculaire [tricuspid endocarditis with right-left shunt in the atrium]. Archives des Maladies du Coeur et des Vaisseaux. 1986;**79**(4):511-513

[15] Szirt R, Youssef GS. Acute right to left shunt-combination of tricuspid valve endocarditis, Chiari network, and ostium

secundum atrial septal defect. Journal of Cardiology Cases. 2017;**16**(5):151-153

[16] Kilit C et al. Double-valve infective endocarditis complicated by a ruptured sinus of Valsalva aneurysm. The American Journal of Cardiology. 2017; **119**:e151. DOI: 10.1016/j.amjcard.2017.03.151

[17] Li JS, Sexton DJ, Mick N, et al. Proposed modifications to the Duke criteria for the diagnosis of infective endocarditis. Clinical Infectious Diseases. 2000;**30**(4):633-638

[18] Bayliss R, Clarke C, Oakley CM, Somerville W, Whitfield AG, Young SE. The microbiology and pathogenesis of infective endocarditis. British Heart Journal. 1983;**50**(6):513-519

[19] Delahaye F, M'Hammedi A, Guerpillon B, et al. Systematic search for present and potential portals of entry for infective endocarditis. Journal of the American College of Cardiology. 2016; **67**(2):151-158

[20] Del Giudice P. Cutaneous complications of intravenous drug abuse. The British Journal of Dermatology. 2004;**150**(1):1-10

[21] Haojun A, Ji Z, Wang Z, et al. Prognostic values of serum procalcitonin and C-reactive protein levels in infective endocarditis. International Journal of Clinical and Experimental Medicine. 2018;**11**(10):10896-10902

[22] Kocazeybek B, Küçükoğlu S, Oner YA. Procalcitonin and C-reactive protein in infective endocarditis: Correlation with etiology and prognosis. Chemotherapy. 2003;**49**(1–2):76-84

[23] Watkin RW, Harper LV, Vernallis AB, et al. Pro-inflammatory cytokines IL6, TNF-alpha, IL1beta, procalcitonin, lipopolysaccharide binding protein and C-reactive protein in infective endocarditis. The Journal of Infection. 2007;**55**(3):220-225

[24] Huang S, Zhou Z, Luo L, et al. Preoperative serum albumin: A promising indicator of early mortality after surgery for infective endocarditis. Annals of Translational Medicine. 2021; **9**(18):1445

[25] Ulldemolins M, Roberts JA, Rello J, Paterson DL, Lipman J. The effects of hypoalbuminaemia on optimizing antibacterial dosing in critically ill patients. Clinical Pharmacokinetics. 2011;**50**(2):99-110

[26] Cockerill FR 3rd, Wilson JW, Vetter EA, et al. Optimal testing parameters for blood cultures. Clinical Infectious Diseases. 2004;**38**(12): 1724-1730

[27] Tattevin P, Watt G, Revest M, Arvieux C, Fournier PE. Update on blood culture-negative endocarditis. Médecine et Maladies Infectieuses. 2015; **45**(1–2):1-8

[28] Godfrey R, Curtis S, Schilling WH, James PR. Blood culture negative endocarditis in the modern era of 16S rRNA sequencing. Clinical Medicine (London, England). 2020;**20**(4):412-416

[29] Habib G, Erba PA, Iung B, et al. Clinical presentation, aetiology and outcome of infective endocarditis. Results of the ESC-EORP EURO-ENDO (European infective endocarditis) registry: A prospective cohort study, [published correction appears in Eur Heart J. 2020;41(22):2091]. European Heart Journal. 2019;**40**(39):3222-3232

[30] Siciliano RF, Gualandro DM, Sejas ONE, et al. Outcomes in patients with fungal endocarditis: A multicenter

observational cohort study. International Journal of Infectious Diseases. 2018;**77**: 48-52

[31] Theel ES, Doern CD. β-D-glucan testing is important for diagnosis of invasive fungal infections. Journal of Clinical Microbiology. 2013;**51**(11): 3478-3483

[32] Gómez-Núñez N, Vargas-Barrón J, Espinola-Zavaleta N, et al. Echocardiographic study of patients with congenital heart disease and infective endocarditis. Echocardiography. 2001; **18**(6):485-490

[33] Greaves K, Mou D, Patel A, Celermajer DS. Clinical criteria and the appropriate use of transthoracic echocardiography for the exclusion of infective endocarditis. Heart. 2003; **89**(3):273-275

[34] Evangelista A, Gonzalez-Alujas MT. Echocardiography in infective endocarditis. Heart. 2004;**90**(6):614-617

[35] San Román JA, Vilacosta I, Zamorano JL, Almería C, Sánchez-Harguindey L. Transesophageal echocardiography in right-sided endocarditis. Journal of the American College of Cardiology. 1993;**21**(5): 1226-1230

[36] Sengupta PP, Khandheria BK. Transoesophageal echocardiography. Heart. 2005;**91**(4):541-547

[37] Pedersen WR, Walker M, Olson JD, et al. Value of transesophageal echocardiography as an adjunct to transthoracic echocardiography in evaluation of native and prosthetic valve endocarditis. Chest. 1991;**100**(2):351-356

[38] Habib G, Lancellotti P, Antunes MJ, et al. 2015 ESC guidelines for the management of infective endocarditis: The task force for the Management of Infective Endocarditis of the European Society of Cardiology (ESC). Endorsed by: European Association for Cardio-Thoracic Surgery (EACTS), the European Association of Nuclear Medicine (EANM). European Heart Journal. 2015;**36**(44):3075-3128

[39] Baddour LM, Wilson WR, Bayer AS, et al. Infective endocarditis in adults: Diagnosis, antimicrobial therapy, and Management of Complications: A scientific statement for healthcare professionals from the American Heart Association. Circulation. 2015;**132**(15): 1435-1486

[40] Ten Hove D, Slart RHJA, Sinha B, Glaudemans AWJM, Budde RPJ. 18F-FDG PET/CT in infective endocarditis: Indications and approaches for standardization. Current Cardiology Reports. 2021;**23**(9):130

[41] Swart LE, Gomes A, Scholtens AM, et al. Improving the diagnostic performance of 18F-Fluorodeoxyglucose positron-emission tomography/ computed tomography in prosthetic heart valve endocarditis. Circulation. 2018;**138**(14):1412-1427

[42] Erba PA, Sollini M, Conti U, et al. Radiolabeled WBC scintigraphy in the diagnostic workup of patients with suspected device-related infections. JACC: Cardiovascular Imaging. 2013; **6**(10):1075-1086

[43] Auckenthaler RW. Laboratory diagnosis of infective endocarditis. European Heart Journal. 1984;**5** (Suppl. C):49-51

[44] Nakhleh RE. Quality in surgical pathology communication and reporting. Archives of Pathology & Laboratory Medicine. 2011;**135**(11):1394-1397

[45] Karcioglu ZA. A problem that is older than the hills: The communication gap between the pathologist and the surgeon. Ocular Oncology and Pathology. 2020;**6**(1):1-2

[46] Habib G, Badano L, Tribouilloy C, et al. Recommendations for the practice of echocardiography in infective endocarditis. European Journal of Echocardiography. 2010;**11**(2): 202-219

[47] Shmueli H, Thomas F, Flint N, Setia G, Janjic A, Siegel RJ. Right-sided infective endocarditis 2020: Challenges and updates in diagnosis and treatment. Journal of the American Heart Association. 2020;**9**(15): e017293

[48] Otto CM, Nishimura RA, Bonow RO, et al. 2020 ACC/AHA guideline for the Management of Patients with Valvular Heart Disease: Executive summary: A report of the American College of Cardiology/ American Heart Association joint committee on clinical practice guidelines. Circulation. 2021;**143**(5): e35-e71

[49] Prendergast BD, Tornos P. Surgery for infective endocarditis: Who and when? Circulation. 2010;**121**(9): 1141-1152

[50] Norman G, Atkinson RA, Smith TA, et al. Intracavity lavage and wound irrigation for prevention of surgical site infection. Cochrane Database of Systematic Reviews. 2017;**10**(10): CD012234

[51] Fowler JR, Perkins TA, Buttaro BA, Truant AL. Bacteria adhere less to barbed monofilament than braided sutures in a contaminated wound model. Clinical Orthopaedics and Related Research. 2013;**471**(2):665-671

[52] Belluschi I, Del Forno B, Lapenna E, et al. Surgical techniques for tricuspid valve disease. Frontiers in Cardiovascular Medicine. 2018;**5**:118

[53] Calafiore A, Di Mauro M. Tricuspid valve repair—Indications and techniques: Suture annuloplasty and band annuloplasty. Operative Techniques in Thoracic and Cardiovascular Surgery. 2011;**16**(2): 86-96

[54] Vincent JL. Metabolic support in sepsis and multiple organ failure: More questions than answers. Critical Care Medicine. 2007;**35**(9 Suppl): S436-S440

[55] Wischmeyer PE. Nutrition therapy in sepsis. Critical Care Clinics. 2018; **34**(1):107-125

[56] Fedoruk LM, Jamieson WR, Ling H, et al. Predictors of recurrence and reoperation for prosthetic valve endocarditis after valve replacement surgery for native valve endocarditis. The Journal of Thoracic and Cardiovascular Surgery. 2009;**137**(2): 326-333

[57] Urbandt P, Santana O, Mihos CG, Pineda AM, Lamelas J. Minimally invasive approach for isolated tricuspid valve surgery. The Journal of Heart Valve Disease. 2014;**23**(6):783-787

[58] Münster K, Andersen U, Mikkelsen J, Pettersson G. Vacuum assisted venous drainage (VAVD). Perfusion. 1999;**14**(6):419-423

[59] Shin H, Mori M, Matayoshi T, Suzuki R, Yozu R. Resection of giant right atrial lymphoma using vacuum-assisted cardiopulmonary bypass without snaring the inferior vena cava. Annals of Thoracic and Cardiovascular Surgery. 2004;**10**(4):249-251

[60] Boodram S, Evans E. Use of leukocyte-depleting filters during cardiac surgery with cardiopulmonary bypass: A review. The Journal of Extra-Corporeal Technology. 2008;**40**(1):27-42

[61] Diab M, Platzer S, Guenther A, et al. Assessing efficacy of CytoSorb haemoadsorber for prevention of organ dysfunction in cardiac surgery patients with infective endocarditis: REMOVE-protocol for randomised controlled trial. BMJ Open. 2020;**10**(3):e031912

[62] Arbulu A, Holmes RJ, Asfaw I. Tricuspid valvulectomy without replacement. Twenty years' experience. The Journal of Thoracic and Cardiovascular Surgery. 1991;**102**(6): 917-922

[63] Arbulu A. Trivalvular/bivalvular heart: A philosophical, scientific and therapeutic concept. The Journal of Heart Valve Disease. 2000;**9**(3):353-358

[64] Anil Kumar V, Francis E, Sreehari S, Raj B. Tricuspid valve mycetoma in an infant successfully treated by excision and complex tricuspid valve repair followed by fluconazole therapy. Surgical Infections. 2014;**15**(2):134-140

[65] Anderson JR, Scott P, Nair RU. Conservative surgery in multiple cusp involvement in tricuspid valve endocarditis. British Heart Journal. 1991; **66**(3):244-245

[66] Brescia AA, Watt TMF, Williams AM, Romano MA, Bolling SF. Tricuspid valve leaflet repair and augmentation for infective endocarditis. Operative Techniques in Thoracic and Cardiovascular Surgery. 2019;**24**(4): 206-218

[67] Kluin J, Sojak V, Koolbergen DR, Boon R, Bökenkamp R, Hazekamp MG. Fifteen years' experience with the use of artificial chords for valve reconstruction in children. European Journal of Cardio-Thoracic Surgery. 2017;**52**(6): 1155-1160

[68] Chang BC, Song SW, Lee S, Yoo KJ, Kang MS, Chung N. Eight-year outcomes of tricuspid annuloplasty using autologous pericardial strip for functional tricuspid regurgitation. The Annals of Thoracic Surgery. 2008;**86**(5): 1485-1493

[69] Lee H, Kim J, Oh SS, Yoo JS. Long-term clinical and hemodynamic outcomes of edge-to-edge repair for tricuspid regurgitation. The Annals of Thoracic Surgery. 2021 Sep;**112**(3): 803-808

[70] Sarraj A, Duarte J. Adjustable segmental tricuspid annuloplasty: A new modified technique. The Annals of Thoracic Surgery. 2007;**83**(2):698-699

[71] Ghanta RK, Chen R, Narayanasamy N, et al. Suture bicuspidization of the tricuspid valve versus ring annuloplasty for repair of functional tricuspid regurgitation: Midterm results of 237 consecutive patients. The Journal of Thoracic and Cardiovascular Surgery. 2007;**133**(1): 117-126

[72] Lurz P, Stephan von Bardeleben R, Weber M, et al. Transcatheter edge-to-edge repair for treatment of tricuspid regurgitation. Journal of the American College of Cardiology. 2021;**77**(3): 229-239

[73] Mestres CA, Castellá M, Moreno A, et al. Cryopreserved mitral homograft in the tricuspid position for infective endocarditis: A valve that can be repaired in the long-term (13 years). The Journal of Heart Valve Disease. 2006; **15**(3):389-391

[74] Luciani GB, de Manna ND, Segreto A, Lanzoni L, Faggian G. Scalloped freehand pulmonary homograft for prosthetic tricuspid valve replacement. The Annals of Thoracic Surgery. 2021;**112**(1):e61-e64

[75] Couetil JP, Argyriadis PG, Shafy A, et al. Partial replacement of the tricuspid valve by mitral homografts in acute endocarditis. The Annals of Thoracic Surgery. 2002;**73**(6):1808-1812

[76] Cardarelli MG, Gammie JS, Brown JM, Poston RS, Pierson RN 3rd, Griffith BP. A novel approach to tricuspid valve replacement: The upside down stentless aortic bioprosthesis. The Annals of Thoracic Surgery. 2005;**80**(2): 507-510

[77] Reineke DC, Roost E, Schoenhoff F, et al. Transcatheter treatment of tricuspid valve disease: An unmet need? The surgical point of view. Frontiers in Cardiovascular Medicine. 2018;**5**:98

[78] Renzulli A, De Feo M, Carozza A, et al. Surgery for tricuspid valve endocarditis: A selective approach. Heart and Vessels. 1999;**14**(4):163-169

[79] Arbulu A, Holmes RJ, Asfaw I. Surgical treatment of intractable right-sided infective endocarditis in drug addicts: 25 years experience. The Journal of Heart Valve Disease. 1993;**2**(2): 129-139

[80] Akinosoglou K, Apostolakis E, Koutsogiannis N, Leivaditis V, Gogos CA. Right-sided infective endocarditis: Surgical management. European Journal of Cardio-Thoracic Surgery. 2012;**42**(3):470-479

[81] Carozza A, Renzulli A, De Feo M, et al. Tricuspid repair for infective endocarditis: Clinical and echocardiographic results. Texas Heart Institute Journal. 2001;**28**(2):96-101

[82] Ren ZY, Shi J, Epstein DH, Wang J, Lu L. Abnormal pain response in pain-sensitive opiate addicts after prolonged abstinence predicts increased drug craving. Psychopharmacology. 2009; **204**(3):423-429

[83] Edelstein S, Yahalom M. Cardiac device-related endocarditis: Epidemiology, pathogenesis, diagnosis and treatment - a review. International Journal of Angiology. 2009;**18**(4): 167-172

[84] Klug D, Balde M, Pavin D, et al. Risk factors related to infections of implanted pacemakers and cardioverter-defibrillators: Results of a large prospective study. Circulation. 2007; **116**(12):1349-1355

[85] Nery PB, Fernandes R, Nair GM, et al. Device-related infection among patients with pacemakers and implantable defibrillators: Incidence, risk factors, and consequences. Journal of Cardiovascular Electrophysiology. 2010;**21**(7):786-790

[86] Sohail MR, Henrikson CA, Braid-Forbes MJ, Forbes KF, Lerner DJ. Mortality and cost associated with cardiovascular implantable electronic device infections. Archives of Internal Medicine. 2011;**171**(20):1821-1828

[87] Greenspon AJ, Patel JD, Lau E, et al. 16-year trends in the infection burden for pacemakers and implantable cardioverter-defibrillators in the United States 1993 to 2008. Journal of the American College of Cardiology. 2011; **58**(10):1001-1006

[88] Mahmood M, Kendi AT, Farid S, et al. Role of 18F-FDG PET/CT in the diagnosis of cardiovascular implantable

electronic device infections: A meta-analysis. Journal of Nuclear Cardiology. 2019;**26**(3):958-970

[89] Ahmed FZ, Arumugam P. 18F-FDG PET/CT now endorsed by guidelines across all types of CIED infection: Evidence limited but growing. Journal of Nuclear Cardiology. 2019;**26**(3):971-974

[90] Love CJ. Lead management and Lead extraction. Cardiac Electrophysiology Clinics. 2018;**10**(1): 127-136

[91] Korantzopoulos P, Sideris S, Dilaveris P, Gatzoulis K, Goudevenos JA. Infection control in implantation of cardiac implantable electronic devices: Current evidence, controversial points, and unresolved issues. Europace. 2016; **18**(4):473-478

[92] Woodard DA, Kim G, Nilsson KR. Risk profiles and outcomes of patients receiving antibacterial cardiovascular implantable electronic device envelopes: A retrospective analysis. World Journal of Cardiology. 2022;**14**(3):177-186

[93] Kang FG, Liu PJ, Liang LY, et al. Effect of pocket irrigation with antimicrobial on prevention of pacemaker pocket infection: A meta-analysis. BMC Cardiovascular Disorders. 2017;**17**(1):256

[94] Chirillo F, Scotton P, Rocco F, et al. Impact of a multidisciplinary management strategy on the outcome of patients with native valve infective endocarditis. The American Journal of Cardiology. 2013;**112**(8):1171-1176

Chapter 4

Injection Drug Use-Associated Infective Endocarditis

Erin Barnes and Julia Cook

Abstract

Injection drug use-associated presents is a unique entity. The demographics of those affected and the clinical presentation are markedly different from those with endocarditis due to other causes. This group presents with a high proportion of right sided valve involvement, distinct pathophysiology, and a more varied array of infectious causes. The best management of these patients regarding medications and surgery remain hotly contested. The increased use of oral antibiotics and novel treatment techniques may expand safe and effective treatment for this group of patients.

Keywords: endocarditis, epidemiology, persons who inject drugs, drug use, endocarditis treatment

1. Introduction

Injection drug use (IDU) has long been recognized as a risk factor for endocarditis with case reports of endocarditis in persons who inject drugs (PWID) dating back at least to the 1930s [1]. Injection drug use-associated infected endocarditis (IDU-IE) presents with a relatively unique clinical presentation, is associated with a wide variety of antimicrobial pathogens, and presents multiple practical and ethical challenges to providing effective treatment. We review in this chapter the epidemiology of IDU and resulting IDU-IE in various aspects of the globe. We then further assess the pathophysiology, clinical presentation, microbiology, and management strategies for effective IDU-IE treatment. We end with a brief review of novel approaches to treatment including treatment of the underlying substance use disorder.

2. Injection drug use and IDU-IE across the globe

The epidemiology of IDU-IE generally reflects that of all PWID in a given time and place. It is notoriously difficult to determine the prevalence of IDU in a given population due to the hidden nature of drug use. Measures are most limited outside of Europe, Asia, North America and Australia. With these limitations noted, it is estimated that 11 million persons injected drugs worldwide in 2019 [2]. Central Asia has higher rates of PWID than other parts of Asia but it is less populous than other parts of the Asian Continent. Therefore more than a quarter of all PWID are estimated to reside in East and Southeast Asia, at least 3–5 million persons [3]. A high rate of HIV

IntechOpen

co-infection in PWID in Asia has resulted in overlapping syndemics. The proportion of females is highly variable with estimates ranging from only 3% in South Asia to 20.8% in East and Southeast Asia [3].

Europe has seen a progressive decline in IDU throughout the 2010s [4]. There is a wide range of prevalence of PWID in Europe with the lowest rates estimated in the countries of Belgium, Greece, Spain, Hungary, and the Netherlands. Eastern Europe has a larger proportion of PWID than Western Europe. Heroin is the predominant drug injected though stimulants and other medications are occasionally injected as well. Czechia reports a particularly high rate of methamphetamine-associated injection drug use compared to other European countries. An estimated 25–28% of PWID are women in Europe which is slightly lower than North America and Australia at 30 and 33% respectively [3, 5, 6].

The United States has seen a dramatic rise in IDU as part of an ongoing opioid epidemic. The FDA began fast-tracking opioid drug applications in the early 1990s and the Pain As a 5th Vital Sign™ campaign requiring frequent assessment, scaling and treatment of pain launched in 1995 [7, 8]. In 1996 the juggernaut Oxycontin® was unleashed by Purdue Pharma [9] with employed physicians to spread the message of 'safe yet effective' pain relief to other physicians by citing the 1% addiction rate from an out of context, single paragraph NEJM letter [10]. It gave away millions of coupons for free samples, and netted itself 1 billion in sales annually by 2001 [9, 11]. Opioid use increased 1448% from 1996 to 2011 [12] and in 2012 the CDC declared prescription opioid overdose a national epidemic [13] with reported increases in hepatitis C, hepatitis B, and IDU-IE shortly following. Substance use disorders proceeded to rise in populations who were disproportionately prescribed prescription opioids including rural populations [14] and women [15]. By the 2010s women had gone from approximately 20% of regular opioid users to 50% [16]. The opioid epidemic in the US has since shifted from the original prescription opioid predominance to heroin, synthetic fentanyl analogs, and co-administration of stimulants. These shifts have resulted in large increases in rates of substance use disorder and overdose in men (approximately 2.5 times the rate of women in 2019), racial minorities, and large urban settings [17, 18].

The overall incidence of endocarditis in PWID, though difficult to assess, is much higher than average. One study estimates up to 11.9 cases per 100,000 person years [19] in comparison to 1.4–6.2 cases per 100,000 person years in the general population [20]. Another estimate places the rate closer to 20-times that of the general population [21]. A recent international prospective endocarditis study found that among 11 centers sampled in the US with >500 IE cases, about 16% were IDU-related [20]. Europe and Asian Countries had about 9% associated with active intravenous drug use while South American had <1%. Slipczuk's systematic review complements these findings of a statistically significant increase in reported IDU-related cases in N. America from 17.3% in the 1980s to 50.7% in the 2000s consistent with the above noted rise in PWID due to the US opioid epidemic [22]. Meanwhile the rates of IDU-IE decreased in Europe in the early 2000s from 21.1% in the 1990s to 6.8%, $p < 0.01$). A recent Swedish study found a decrease in cases beginning in 2011 [23]. General IE is reported to affect males in 60–70% of cases [24] but there is a lack of systematic study on gender in IDU-IE. Studies performed since 2000 in the US generally have reported females as 30–55% of the patient population [25–27] which would be similar to slightly higher than the estimated proportion of females who inject drugs in North America. Further study is needed to determine the relative risk of endocarditis in male versus female PWID.

3. Right sided endocarditis in persons who inject drugs

Endocarditis of the tricuspid and pulmonic valves, or right-sided infective endocarditis (RSIE), is rarer than left-sided endocarditis and is classically cited as occurring in 5–10% of all IE cases [28]. Risk factors include IDU along with healthcare associated devices such as cardiac implants, hemodialysis catheters, and other long term venous access devices. The exact proportion of RSIE in PWID presenting with IE is difficult to determine as most reports on this topic are single center and/or retrospective in nature. In the late 1940s and 1950s, reports first began to be published of endocarditis in PWID making note of markedly higher proportions of tricuspid valve (TV) endocarditis and S. aureus involvement [29]. This phenomenon was met with scrutiny. A relatively large series by Cherubin et al. from 1960 to 1967 of 36 IDU-IE cases had TV involvement in 18% (9% sole TV, 9% in combination with another valve) [30]. While acknowledging that this is still larger than the 5–10% of TV cases seen in the non-injecting population, the authors proposed that the increased frequency of TV reports were due to either reporting bias or regional variation in drug use as many of the previous cases reported were from the Washington DC area [30]. Since this original debate in the literature many reports have gone on to find TV valve predominance in IDU-IE cases [31–40], but not all [27, 41–47]. The reasons for these differences and their meaning remain unclear. Some study populations are surgical populations which may bias towards left-sided disease. Studies in the 1980s through mid-1990s predominately were in HIV positive patients which may have confounded presentation. At least one study has suggested that the substance of use may influence the phenotype of endocarditis [48]. Within these limitations, all that can be said with certainty is that right sided-endocarditis remains over-represented in this population but left-sided endocarditis is also commonplace.

The pathology of RSIE is still not fully understood. The right side of the heart has lower pressures than the left and the valves are thus less prone to sclerosis and injury of the endothelium associated with high biomechanical forces. Injury to the endothelium of the right heart valves likely occurs through distinct mechanisms in IDU-IE. Some substances are directly toxic to endothelial cells and cardiomyocytes, particularly stimulants such as cocaine [49]. Particulate damage also plays a role. Most injected substances begin as powders or pills and may not fully dissolve in solution. Particulate matter is injected along with substances which bombards and disrupts the endothelium of the right heart before being filtered out by the lungs. Evidence suggests this is particularly true for pills which are crushed and injected with multiple reports of talc granulomas found within the lungs and heart valves of PWID [50, 51]. PWID are themselves aware of the potential damage from particulate matter and use a variety of devices ranging from medical grade filters to cigarette filters to strain their drugs; in many places filters are a provided as a component of harm reduction [52, 53]. There are no studies on whether filter use by PWID limits risk of IDU-IE.

Endothelium is naturally resistant to infection and even when damaged, only certain types and strains of bacteria with particular virulence factors can bind [54–58]. As bacteria adhere and invade, our immune system activates in an attempt to repair the damage and remove invaders. This results in an amalgam of fibrin and platelets being deposited in the area along with the bacteria resulting in a bacterial vegetation. An alternative sequence of vegetation formation involves the repair of injured valve endothelium by fibrin and platelets which form a sterile vegetation later seeded by a bacteremia. Indeed, some pathogens may lack virulence factors which would allow them to bind directly to the damaged endothelium but which facilitate binding to the matrix of nonbacterial thrombotic lesions [58]. Regardless of event sequence, as this vegetation of platelets, fibrin, and bacteria grow the vegetation acts as a physical barrier protecting the embedded pathogens from immune regulation [59]. In addition, organisms at the center of the vegetation are concentrated at a higher density with fewer resources and go into a restricted growth phase which impairs the ability of antibiotics to eradicate them [60]. Finally, the nutrition deficiencies experienced by these deeper organisms that have been present longest in the vegetation develop morphological changes in cell wall thickness and increase their excretion of polysaccharides to form biofilms which further alter antibiotic susceptibility [61].

The distinctive pathophysiology of right-sided endocarditis combined with the low pressure, low biomechanical stress environment of right-sided vascular endothelium combine to alter the characteristics and risks of the endocarditis vegetation. The left-sided endocarditis literature tends to identify vegetations greater than 1 centimeter as being at increased risk of embolization and poor outcome [62]. This makes intuitive sense as a larger vegetation would be more friable while also being more subject to forces propelling it form the valve. However on the right side of the heart, vegetations measuring 2 to 3 cm are regularly described and the correlation between size and clinical outcomes is less clear [63, 64]. Vegetations ≥2 cm on right sided valves have been suggested to correlate with increased all cause mortality [63, 65] but evidence for this conclusion remains limited. Some of the lowered mortality for large vegetations in RSIE is due to the fact that unless a patent foramen ovale is present the vegetations embolize to the lung rather than the CNS; embolization to the CNS is an independent predictor of poor outcome. Another mitigating factor is the lower likelihood of heart failure with compromised right sided heart valves compared to left.

RSIE is more easily diagnosed by transthoracic echocardiogram (TTE) as the right-sided structures are located more anterior with a shorter distance between the transducer and structures [28]. Transesophageal echocardiography (TEE) is still superior to TTE for RSIE related to cardiac devices and has increased sensitivity for small vegetations and annular abscess. Endocarditis of the pulmonic valve or eustachian valve is also better visualized on TEE [28]. European and American guidelines indicate that TEE is not mandatory in isolated, native-valve, RSIE when TTE images are of high quality and risk of complication is low [62, 66]. In cases where TTE and TEE are unrevealing but high clinical suspicion remains, more advanced imaging techniques may be considered including 18F-fluorodeoxyglucose positron emission tomography/CT, cardiac CT, or radiolabeled white blood cells scintigraphy. This field of study continues to involve but studies indicated that these methods may have increased sensitivity in instances such as prosthetic infections and have the additional benefit of identifying silent emboli and aneurysms [66].

4. Population specific considerations

4.1 Women

Women who use drugs are more likely than men to develop clinical addiction and more rapidly progress to severe addiction [67]. Among those who seek treatment, women have higher opioid craving scores [68], psychiatric comorbidities [69], and physical health problems than their male counterparts [69, 70]. Given these differences, it is not surprising that women may also use their drugs differently.

Some studies have shown women are more likely to inject their preferred substance of abuse [71], are more likely to share needles and equipment [72], and possibly inject more frequently than males [73]. These behaviors increase infectious risk, including for IDU-IE. A retrospective study found that among HIV positive PWID, females had higher odds of IE with a multivariate OR of 3.26 (95% CI 1·73–6·14) [34]. A second study with 17 cases of IDU-IE found a similar trend but did not reach statistical significance (OR 1·62, 95% CI 0·61–4·34) [74]. Smaller/deeper veins resulting in more tissue damage during injection has been one theory proposed to explain this finding [34]. Another is the possibility for more rapid sclerosis of their smaller peripheral veins resulting in migration to high risk injection sites such as the jugular vein [75].

4.2 HIV population

HIV and endocarditis have overlapping risk factors and there are multiple studies assessing the outcomes of endocarditis in HIV positive persons. Early in the HIV epidemic it was feared that the cardiopulmonary bypass required for surgery could hasten the advancement to AIDS as a result of the general immunosuppression observed after major surgical procedures in combination with general anesthesia [76]. In the era of combined highly active antiretroviral therapy, studies indicate no worse outcomes in HIV positive patients requiring cardiac surgery compared to the general population [77]. A study by Ortega et al. in Spain found that the incidence of IDU-IE in persons living with HIV decreased with the advent of highly active antiretroviral therapy [78]. HIV does not seem to worsen the outcomes of IE unless severe immunosuppression is present with an AIDS defining condition and/or CD4+ cell counts <200/microL [79, 80]. A general trend corresponding to increased mortality with declining CD4+ count below 500 microL has been observed [81].

5. Endocarditis pathogens in persons who inject drugs

PWID have been found to have endocarditis with a wide variety of pathogens. Some atypical pathogens have been reported to be more common in this population due to a variety of factors including varied skin colonization patterns, risk imposed by the substances themselves, or through the agents used as solvents.

5.1 Methicillin resistant staphylococcus aureus (MRSA)

Staphylococcus aureus has been found to be the most common endocarditis pathogen in many industrialized countries but this shift with Staphylococcal predominance was first noted in those with IDU-IE [24]. S. aureus remains the most common pathogen implicated in IDU-IE [82]. PWID are estimated to be 16.3 times as likely to develop invasive MRSA infections that others. In a recent study assessing surveillance data from 6 sites across the US, the proportion of invasive MRSA cases that occurred among PWIDs increased from 4.1% in 2011 to 9.2% in 2016. Of these cases, 20% were IE [83]. Studies indicate that people who are colonized with S. aureus are at higher risk of infection [84] and additional studies indicate that PWID have high rates of colonization [84]. When they develop clinical infections with S. aureus it is with the specific strains with which they are colonized [85]. The exact mechanism for increased colonization and infection by MRSA in PWID is unclear. It may be that the nature of shared drug use environments, crowded and unsanitary conditions, and frequent healthcare center exposures may lead to transmission of S. aureus in this community [86]. Repetitive disruption of the skin barrier can then enable deep seated infections including IDU-IE.

Right-sided disease accounts for about 66% of IDU-associated S. aureus endocarditis [87, 88]. There are also studies that show a relatively high rate of multivalve S. aureus infection compared to people who do not inject drugs [87]. The mortality rate of S. aureus endocarditis in PWID is lower than in people who do not inject drugs which is thought to be due to younger age and fewer comorbid conditions [39, 87, 89, 90]. Embolic events generally occur at a higher rate with S. aureus IE compared with IE due to other pathogens [91, 92]. Studies usually report a lower rate of surgery for PWID with S. aureus IE than in people who do not inject drugs. Current treatment guidelines recommend treating S. aureus associated endocarditis with 6 weeks of therapy [62].

5.2 Candida

IE due to candida species is relatively rare, accounting for around 2–4% of all cases [93, 94]. Multiple outbreaks of disseminated candida infections have been traced back to using lemon juice as a solvent for intravenous heroin and cocaine [95–97]. Acids such as lemon juice are commonly used to dissolve brown heroin, which is a base form less water soluble than the white, salt form of heroin. Similarly the crack form of cocaine is prepared for injection with the addition of an acid [98]. Lemon juice has been shown to readily grow Candida at room temperature, and the belief is that the resultant infection is due to injection of a high inoculum of Candida by PWID [95]. These disseminated candida infections have a predilection for endogenous spread to the eye, with resultant endophthalmitis in addition to endocarditis. Sterile packages of ascorbic acid are provided in many harm reduction centers to minimize the risk of Candida infections. Current treatment guidelines for native valve Candida IE recommend initial management with lipid formulation amphotericin B with or without flucytosine or a high dose echinocandin. This is then followed by step-down therapy with an azole. Valve replacement is recommended, and long term suppression is recommended for patients who cannot undergo valve replacement followed by chronic suppression [62].

5.3 Non-HACEK gram negatives

Compared to the general population, PWID are at increased risk of non-HACEK gram negative endocarditis though this is still a rare clinical entity [99, 100]. A recent single center study from the southeast US identified 43 cases of gram negative IE, of which 93% had a history of or active injection drug use [101]. In other recent studies nosocomial acquisition was a more common risk factor than IDU [100, 102]. In the US study the majority of these patients had had a prior instance of IE and most cases were of native valves, predominately right-sided valves. Of these cases, 68% were associated with Pseudomonas aeruginosa, 20% Serratia marcescens, and the remaining were with Enterobacter cloacae, Klebsiella oxytoca, and Acinetobacter baumannii. These patients were very ill, with 60% requiring a stay in the intensive care unit during their hospitalization and roughly 25% underwent valve surgery; the 12 month all-cause mortality rate was 30%. This is consistent with the overall 20–30% mortality seen in IE caused by non-HACEK gram negative bacilli though this mortality rate encompasses a wide range of patient populations with many having multiple underlying comorbidities [103].

Pseudomonas is one of the most common non-HACEK organisms cited in this group [104]. The major source of Pseudomonas IE appears to be contaminated water used to mix drugs for injection and this may explain the presence of other water organisms such as S. marcescens as well [105, 106]. In a Pseudomonal endocarditis outbreak in Detroit occurring in the 1970s–1980s associated with injection of dissolved pentazocine and tripelennamine('Ts and blues'), the drug itself was found to act as a selective culture medium which inhibited the growth of S. aureus and many pseudomonas strains but not serotype O11 strains which were associated with the invasive infections [107]. S. marcescens is increasingly being reported in US literature as well though the exact association or cause of this increase remains unclear [106, 108]. One factor that may select for gram negatives in this group is intensive or frequent therapy for gram positive bacteria that cause skin abscesses and more frequent deep-seated infections thus resulting in selective pressure. Evidence for this is found in the high rate of gram negative bacilli (and Candida) blood stream infections found in persons who continued to inject while on therapy for predominately gram positive infections [109]. Evidence for management of infections by these organisms is limited and current treatment guidelines recommend consideration of surgical management in addition to dual antibiotic therapy for 6 weeks. Proposed combinations are a beta-lactam in combination with either a fluoroquinolone or aminoglycoside [62].

5.4 Others

There are innumerable case reports describing unusual pathogens isolated in this patient population, frequently in the setting of polymicrobial infections [110, 111]. This includes non-tuberculous mycobacteria which should be considered as a possible cause of culture negative endocarditis [112]. Speical blood culture medium is required for acid fast bacteria and they may still be difficult to culture with a long window between collection and resultant growth. Endocarditis secondary to unusual or fastidious oral flora, including Neisseria sicca and anaerobes such as Veillonella sp., have been in described in this population in association with those who lick their needles prior to injection [113, 114]. Given the paucity of treatment evidence for severe infections with these types of organisms and the increased mortality associated with polymicrobial infections, treatment is individualized and outcomes with these types of organisms and infections is frequently higher than average.

6. Treatment difficulties of IDU-IE

6.1 Antibiotic delivery and oral antibiotics

How to best provide prolonged intravenous therapy to PWID is a particularly perplexing issue. Concerns regarding discharge with an intravenous line include potential use of the catheter for drug injection, seeding the line with transient bacteremia even if the line itself is not used to inject, and difficulty finding home health companies for this population. Countries over the world have different outpatient parenteral antibiotic therapy (OPAT) systems and healthcare delivery models making this topic even more difficult to analyze. Antibiotic delivery models include infusion at ambulatory care centers or in the home by home care nurses (more common in European countries) or discharge of patients home to administer their own parenteral antibiotics with only weekly home health oversight (the US). These differing models with variable degrees of patient oversight result in differing risk of discharge of PWID with a central catheter. Some studies have shown OPAT can be done relatively safely in PWID, but these studies contained a large proportion of persons retained in a facility of some type or were noted to require particularly intensive oversight [115]. Given the difficulties and challenges of this group, many health facilities retain their population with IDU-IE inpatient or at an affiliated facility for the duration of their treatment [116]. This strategy is frustrating for patients and uses large amounts of healthcare resources. IDU-IE in the US was recently estimated to have direct costs of $180,000 and cost significantly more than IE attributed to causes other than IDU [117].

For all of these reasons, short course and oral therapy are very attractive options. Studies show that 2 week courses of IV beta-lactam therapy in isolated tricuspid valve IE secondary to methicillin susceptible S. aureus (MSSA) with no embolic phenomena outside of the lungs can be successful. Multiple studies have evaluated this strategy over time predominately with the use of cloxacillin [118]. Addition of an aminoglycoside was not found to significantly alter outcomes in one study though most studies evaluating this short-course strategy evaluated the beta-lactam in combination with an aminoglycoside [119]. These studies were generally performed when co-administration of aminoglycosides was routine and recommended for S aureus IE. This is no longer the case and the most recent American guidelines discourage the use even in right-sided endocarditis [62]. Evidence indicates that the use of a glycopeptide for short course therapy such as would be required for MRSA is not efficacious even when combined with an aminoglycoside [120].

Oral antibiotics offer even greater appeal. In 1989 Dworkin published 14 cases of right sided, S aureus IDU-IE treated with ciprofloxacin and rifampin [121]. Heldman et al. then completed a randomized control trial of oxacillin/gentamicin compared to ciprofloxacin/rifampin in 85 right-sided IDU-IE patients; 41 did not complete therapy and only 44 were analyzed. There were three failures in the standard arm and one in the oral arm. While these results are reassuring, they may not be fully generalizable to today's population. Between these two studies only 15% had pulmonary emboli and only 28% with echocardiograms had visible vegetations. While this may in part reflect limits of older echocardiographic technology, those caring for populations with visible vegetations must be wary. Large vegetations are those which are most difficult to treat due to the organism density and limited antibiotic penetration into vegetations [122–124]. Additionally, only 5% of Heldman's population had MRSA. PWID are more prone to MRSA infections which are likely to be fluoroquinolone-resistant [83, 125].

The most important development is the POET trial which randomized 400 left-sided IE patients to a full course of intravenous therapy or changeover to oral therapy [126]. This study included those with cardiac implantable electronic devices (CIEDs), prosthetic valves, and surgical patients and still found that changing to oral therapy was noninferior to full intravenous courses. Generalizing to our IDU-IE population, however, again requires caution. Fewer than 6% of patients had a vegetation >9 mm at the time of randomization. IDU-IE patients with right-sided disease may be less likely to undergo surgery and have large vegetations. More importantly, this population predominately suffered from streptococcal disease. None of these patients had MRSA and the MSSA was highly susceptible, even to penicillin. Doses used for these regimens were much higher than is typically seen such as using 600 mg PO BID of rifampin. This results in a need to ensure that a patient can orally tolerate the medications and that a way to monitor for toxicities of the oral antibiotics is available including office follow-up and blood tests. For this reason those who were deemed unreliable were excluded and only five PWID were included in this study.

In summary, there is increasing and high grade evidence for the safety and efficacy of oral antibiotics in the treatment of endocarditis including IDU-IE but caveats remain. There is very little data on the safety of oral therapies when vegetations are greater than 1 cm in size or where there is extensive co-occurring embolic phenomena. Parameters to guide the frequency of blood testing for safety monitoring on these regimens is lacking and frequent outpatient blood draws in PWID may be further complicated by venous sclerosis and poor venous access. Evidence on orals for treatment of MRSA IE is lacking. Invasive MRSA infection is more common in PWID so this is of particular relevance to this group [83]. Follow-up publications have noted the mutation of methicillin resistance should not affect the function of non-beta-lactam antibiotics and thus regimens which do not rely on this class of agents should be as effective against MRSA as MSSA [127] but clinicians remain cautious.

It must be noted that while the evidence above provides evidence for the option of oral antibiotics and outpatient treatment, multiple additional factors must be incorporated into clinical decision making. The need for complete adherence to a complex medical regimen and close outpatient follow-up may be inherently problematic in this population. Socioeconomic complications including unstable housing, lack of transportation, and unreliable phone service may make care in the outpatient setting untenable. And then there is the risk of ongoing drug use once discharged. This would not only further impair follow-up but risk renal/hepatic injury while on renally-dosed medications, worsening of the current infection, and possible development of a new suprainfection. Each patient will require nuanced and thoughtful decision-making to determine the best treatment course for an individual and their unique set of factors. This precludes the development of any one 'rule' on how to manage this group and practice is likely to remain heterogeneous across institutions and providers.

6.2 Surgery

Perhaps the most difficult aspect of IDU-IE is weighing the risk–benefit of surgery. This group is relatively young. Bioprosthetic valves avoid the need for anticoagulation but are less durable than mechanical valves resulting in higher rates of repair surgeries over time [128]. The main concern, however, is that the patient will re-infect the heart valve through ongoing substance use. Addiction is a chronic, relapsing disease with heroin relapse rates following simple detox as high as 91% [129]. Ongoing injection drug use raises the risk for prosthetic valve endocarditis which has worse outcomes than native valve endocarditis [130]. What timing, surgical approach, and mitigating factors can identify patients who would individually benefit from surgical rather than medical management remain vastly understudied. Benefits of surgery in isolated tricuspid valve endocarditis are the least-well resolved. These concerns have led to significant debate regarding risk-stratification and performance of cardiac surgery in PWID. With the lack of clear guidelines or risk stratification protocols, there is wide variability in surgical management. Some surgeons are only willing to perform a single heart operation while others mitigate their responses by what kind of SUD treatment was available and attained by the patient [131–133].

To help guide clinical decision making, multiple studies have attempted to provide objective assessment of outcomes for those who undergo surgery for IDU-IE but only a small number have compared the outcomes to a contemporaneous population of routine IE. In the English based literature of the last 2 decades, at least 7 US, 2 Swedish, 1 Czech Republic, 1 Italian, 1 international prospective study, and 2 meta-analyses have been published comparing surgical outcomes in IDU-IE to the general IE population [27, 35, 43–45, 47, 134–140]. These comparisons must be taken with a grain of salt given that the compared groups differ in demographics, valve characteristics and pathogen type while also having very different proportions of pre-existing comorbidities. Surgical selection bias also will play a role in determining the timing and type of surgical intervention within and between groups. With these caveats in mind, all of these studies have come to the same conclusion: the in-patient and 30-day mortality of this population is comparable to or better than those undergoing surgery for non-IDU-IE while longer term mortality appears higher. Thalme et al. found that for those undergoing surgery for left sided IE, PWID had significantly higher mortality in the first 5-years despite comparable to better in-patient mortality; none of the 5 surgical patients in the IDU-IE group were alive at 4 years [35]. Rabkin et al. who assessed 197 surgical endocarditis cases including 64 PWID defined as *ever* having injected drugs [44] found on Cox regression analysis that PWID had lower ten-year survival (41·1% IDU vs. 52% non-IDU, $p = 0{\cdot}03$). Ongoing substance use has been found to be the primary driver of this increased long-term mortality in at least one study [141].

These studies also have come to the same broad conclusion that repeat infective endocarditis is more common in this group though exactly how much more common varies across studies. Thalme found the odds of recurrent endocarditis in PWID was 6-fold higher (12·5 vs. 2·3%, OR 6·07, $p = 0{\cdot}007$, 95% CI 1·55–23·70). This aligns with the findings of Kim et al. who found a propensity score matched HR of 6.2 for reinfection in PWID compared to general IE (95% CI 2·56–15, $p < 0{\cdot}001$). The studies by Kaiser and Shrestha assessed a combined 858 surgically treated IE patients of whom 93 were PWID [43, 45]. Both found significantly higher rates of reinfection in PWID (HR 9·8, 95% CI 2·7–35·3 in Shrestha and 17 vs. 5%, $p = 0{\cdot}03$ in Kaiser) [43, 45].

Descriptions of repeat IDU-IE cases are limited despite being relatively common. It appears that repeat infection occurs relatively quickly. In a study of 87 IDU-IE patients surviving their primary hospital stay, 25·7% developed repeat IE within a median of 257 days [142]. Kim et al. found the median time to reinfection was18·1 months [27]. The microbiology is more varied on repeat endocarditis admissions: whereas 95% of one center's patients had S. aureus as the causative pathogen on their first episode, it accounted for only 54% of cases on the second episode where Candida, Enterococcus, and Streptococcus were more common [142]. Finally, repeat endocarditis predisposes to higher mortality. The ICE found that 20% of all IE patients who suffered a recurrent episode were deceased at 1 year compared to 9% surviving a single episode [143]. This difference seems even more profound for IDU-IE as 36% of those with a repeat case were deceased at 1 year vs. 4% of those with a single episode [142]. It is possible that re-infection is a marker of more severe opioid use disorder which then drives the higher mortality rather than the IE itself but these factors are difficult to disentangle.

Medical research has a long way to go in determining how much benefit an individual with IDU-IE is likely to receive by undergoing surgical rather than medical treatment and how to parse that risk in real time. At this time, surgical thresholds vary across countries, institutions, and individual surgeons but the medical literature strongly suggests that when a patient does undergo surgery, they achieve short term survival comparable to their non-IDU-IE peers. Long term outcomes and what role, if any, they should play in acute surgical decision making are more difficult to parse.

7. Areas of exploration: the future of IDU-IE

Given the difficulties noted above, new strategies for treating this group are urgently needed. Some promise lies in the areas of novel antibiotics, novel surgical approaches, and the rise of more integrated addiction care.

7.1 Lipoglycopeptides

The lipoglycopeptides have a long, lipophilic side chain added onto glycopeptides (the class of vancomycin and teicoplanin). The result is similar bactericidal activity but the more lipophilic side chain anchoring onto the bacterial cell membrane results in increased potency and, potentially, half-life [144]. Telavancin, oritavancin, and dalbavancin are all FDA approved for treatment of complex skin and soft tissue infections and Telavancin additionally is approved for pneumonias. The dosing of telavancin is daily while dalbavancin and oritavancin can be dosed weekly.

Telavancin and Dalbavancin currently have the most promising data for endocarditis. Telavancin has been shown in multiple in vitro studies to be at least as effective as daptomycin and vancomycin [145]. In 2010 telavancin was successfully used to treat right sided, native MRSA endocarditis. The patient remained culture positive after 8 days of vancomycin. He was then changed to telavancin with negative cultures resulting in 24 hours [146]. Since then telavancin has been used to successfully treat MRSA mitral valve endocarditis [147] and VISA CIED endocarditis [148].

Dalbavancin also has endocarditis data [149–151]. In the rabbit IE model it was shown that dalbavancin was 2–4-fold more potent than vancomycin [152]. One of the first human endocarditis case was attempted treatment of MRSA native valve endocarditis in a pregnant PWID. She was treated with vancomycin and then daptomycin 10 mg/kg for the first 26 days. Unfortunately there were two treatment interruptions where the patient left against medical advice; after returning from the second interruption she received a 1 g loading dose of dalbavancin followed by 500 mgs weekly for a total of 4 weeks. Unfortunately, she presented to the hospital 11 days after her final dose with S. aureus bacteremia that was now vancomycin intermediate (MIC 4 mcg/mL) and telavancin resistant. It was hypothesized that increased renal filtration and altered protein binding of pregnancy may have decreased the half-life of the drug leading to subtherapeutic levels.

More positive outcomes were found in a 2 year, retrospective study of 24 IE patients transitioned to dalbavancin after clearing their blood cultures on standard care; three patients were started directly on dalbavancin. Causative organisms included S aureus, streptococci, Enterococcus, Aerococcus, and coagulase-negative Staphylococcus. Drug regimens were a 1 g load with 500 mg weekly thereafter and a 1·5 g load with 1 g twice weekly. Mean duration of administration was 6 weeks but ranged from 1-30 weeks. A patient with E faecalis prosthetic valve infection died of surgical complications and another patient failed treatment. This patient had an MRSA CIED infection which could not be fully removed. The patient received 30 weeks of Dalbavancin but then had breakthrough bacteremia. The breakthrough strain showed small colony variants with a vancomycin MIC of 2 mg/L (up from 1 mg/L).

A similar cohort by Wunsch et al. treated 25 endocarditis cases which included 6 prosthetic valves and 4 CIEDs with a similar pathogen cohort [153]. Patients were switched to dalbavancin after having been treated initially with more routine antimicrobials. Nine of the patients received a single 1.5 g dose while 8 received a dose of 1 g on day 1 followed by 500 mg on day 8. Successful treatment was achieved in 92% of patients. The patient who failed treatment died of sepsis from MSSA IE.

Use in IDU-IE has had mixed results due to the difficulty in maintaining this population in treatment. A study of 9 persons with right sided IDU-IE found that only 3 of the patient completed the pre-defined treatment course [154]. Of those with a successful completed course, 2 received a planned single dose and 1 received a planned 2 doses; 4 of those who failed to complete their course were planned to receive only a single dose which highlights the difficulty. Also the most concerning issue to arise from these studies is the potential for resistance. Both the case of the pregnant female and the CIED infection suggest suboptimal treatment can result in rising MICs for vancomycin as well as the lipoglycopeptides. This could conceivably be a problem in PWID who may not return for their follow-up medication doses.

7.2 Delafloxacin

Delafloxacin is a novel fluoroquinolone marketed by Melinta under the brand name Baxdela currently FDA approved for skin and soft tissue infections. A major limitation of oral therapy for endocarditis noted above is MRSA's frequent resistant to fluoroquinolones. However, delafloxacin currently is estimated to have efficacy against 88% of US MRSA strains [155], including those resistant to other fluoroquinolones. This is due to the fact that delafloxacin binds to both the topoisomerase and gyrase in relatively equal amounts whereas other fluoroquinolones tend to more heavily target one enzyme over the other. The result is a lower likelihood of 2 spontaneous mutations developing and lower risk of resistance [156]. This combined with its relatively unique ability to maintain efficacy in acidic environments [156] may allow it to overcome severe MRSA infections such as endocarditis where other oral agents have failed.

7.3 Bacteriophages

The use of lytic bacteriophages as antibacterial therapy has long been hypothesized but clinical studies are in their infancy [157]. To date few persons have been treated with a bacteriophage and only when all other alternatives had been exhausted. The bacteriophage generally must be matched to the pathogen with some pathogens having resistance and repeated testing to assess for acquired resistance with treatment is recommended [158]. Expanded use of phage therapy holds promise for treatment of resistant microorganisms, difficult to treat microorganisms such as MRSA, and device related infections where biofilm plays a significant role in pathology. Endocarditis with its vegetation could fall into the latter group. At least one animal study shows possible synergistic effect between phages and antibiotics for endocarditis treatment [159] and at least seven persons have received adjunctive phage therapy for endocarditis due to S. aureus [160, 161]. The patient seemed to have ongoing clearance and control of the infection with a negative PET on day 80 however ongoing severe heart failure persisted and the patient ultimately expired. What role the phage therapy played as compared to the antibiotics is undetermined. Phage therapy could provide an attractive alternative for those with IDU-IE as it might allow for effective treatment of larger vegetations thereby further limiting the need for surgery. Heightened efficacy may also allow for shorter treatment courses for this condition. Challenges to progressive study in this particular disease state includes the relative rarity of endocarditis, the rapid progression of most endocarditis cases making interventional studies or the matching of phages to pathogen more logistically complex, and the current reserved use of phages only for patient where no alternatives exist.

7.4 Percutaneous aspiration

Percutaneous aspiration of vegetations from the tricuspid valve has been reported with increasing frequency in the last decade [162, 163]. This procedure is performed by placing the patient on an extracorporeal circulatory circuit through large bore venous drainage and venous return cannulas. Under transesophageal echocardiographic guidance, the vacuum-assisted device is frequently performed with use of the AngioVac system, a product of Angiodynamics, USA. The goals of vegetation aspiration are decreased bacterial load, decreased vegetation size to lower embolic risk and antibiotic failure risk, and possibly to limit progressive damage to the valve and cardiac structures. Patients with vegetations greater than 1 cm in size and outside of criteria used in common oral endocarditis treatment studies may become eligible for oral treatment therapies as compared to intravenous following angiovac debulking which may be associated with decreased length of stay and healthcare costs. Prospective and controlled studies on the benefits and risks of this procedure are not yet available but will hopefully be performed in the coming decade.

7.5 Co-addiction treatment

Substance use disorder is a chronic disease making its stabilization and management in the acute care setting challenging. In many instances the substance use disorder is disregarded while the acute condition is treated resulting in problematic disconnect [164]. The first is that patients can withdraw while in the inpatient setting. This can result in increased risk of leaving against medical advice, ongoing substance use during the hospital stay, and increased conflict between provider and patient [165]. Where specialized addiction professionals are unavailable, hospitalists and internists should be familiar with the medications used to treat substance withdrawal and substance use disorders. This will then allow providers to take full advantage of a potential 'teachable moment'. Facilitating detox from substances and intake to treatment is crucial for long term health. A randomized clinical trial found that those who began medication-assisted therapy with buprenorphine while inpatient were significantly more likely to enter treatment post-discharge (72 vs. 12%, $p < 0{\cdot}001$), be engaged in treatment at 6 months (16·7 vs. 3.0% $p = 0{\cdot}007$), and have less illicit opioid use in the 30 days prior to a 6-month interview (incidence rate ratio 0·6, 95% CI 0·46–0·73, $p < 0{\cdot}01$) [166]. Unfortunately, this same study found no significant difference in injection opioid frequency at 6 months among PWID despite the fact that the odds of injection opioid use were 4·57-times higher on days without buprenorphine than with buprenorphine. The authors hypothesized that this specific group might need higher doses to combat more severe addiction and that the new long-acting injectable buprenorphine may improve outcomes [167]. It is worth noting, that reduction in injection frequency, even without full cessation, is associated with decreased risk for invasive bacterial infection [168].

8. Conclusions

IDU-IE remains a distinct entity that is encountered across the globe. In places such as the US there have been great increases in the incidence and prevalence of this disease. Yet the ideal management of this patient population remains understudied and under debate. Ongoing research to identify which patients have the highest benefit from surgical intervention in RSIE are needed. The use of percutaneous aspiration and novel medication such as the lipoglycopeptides provide alternatives to traditional treatment models with increasing use. Most important of all is the need for progressive integration of addiction care into acute care medical management in order to treat the root cause of IDU-IE and achieve long term positive health outcomes.

Author details

Erin Barnes* and Julia Cook
Atrium Health Wake Forest Baptis, Section on Infectious Diseases, Winston Salem, NC, USA

*Address all correspondence to: ewbarnes@wakehealth.edu

References

[1] Luttgens WF. Endocarditis in main line opium addicts; report on 11 cases. Archives of Internal Medicine. 1949;**83**(6):653-664

[2] U. N. O. o. D. a. C. (UNODC). World Drug Report. 2021. Available from: https://www.unodc.org/res/wdr2021/field/WDR21_Booklet_2.pdf (accessed.

[3] Degenhardt L et al. Global prevalence of injecting drug use and sociodemographic characteristics and prevalence of HIV, HBV, and HCV in people who inject drugs: A multistage systematic review. The Lancet Global Health. 2017;**5**(12). DOI: 10.1016/S2214-109X(17)30375-3

[4] Trends and Developments. European Drug Report 2021. 2021

[5] Degenhardt L et al. Meth/amphetamine use and associated HIV: Implications for global policy and public health. The International Journal on Drug Policy. 2010;**21**(5):347-358. DOI: 10.1016/j.drugpo.2009.11.007

[6] Stone K. Reviewing harm reduction for people who inject drugs in Asia: The necessity for growth. Harm Reduction Journal. 2015;**12**:32. DOI: 10.1186/s12954-015-0066-x

[7] Greene MS, Chambers RA. Pseudoaddiction: Fact or fiction? An investigation of the medical literature. Current Addiction Reports. 2015;**2**(4):310-317. DOI: 10.1007/s40429-015-0074-7

[8] deShazo RD, Johnson M, Eriator I, Rodenmeyer K. Backstories on the US opioid epidemic. Good intentions gone bad, an industry gone rogue, and watch dogs gone to sleep. The American Journal of Medicine. 2018;**131**(6):595-601. DOI: 10.1016/j.amjmed.2017.12.045

[9] Van Zee A. The promotion and marketing of oxycontin: Commercial triumph, public health tragedy. American Journal of Public Health. 2009;**99**(2):221-227. DOI: 10.2105/ajph.2007.131714

[10] Porter J, Jick H. Addiction rare in patients treated with narcotics. The New England Journal of Medicine. 1980;**302**(2):123

[11] United States General Accounting Office. Prescription Drugs: OxyContin abuse and diversion and efforts to address the problem. GAO-04-011. 2003. Available from: 0090-0036 (Print)1541-0048 (Electronic). DOI: 10.2105/ajph.2007.131714

[12] Atluri S, Sudarshan G, Manchikanti L. Assessment of the trends in medical use and misuse of opioid analgesics from 2004 to 2011. Pain Physician. 2014;**17**(2):E119-E128

[13] Paulozzi L, Franklin G, Kerlikowske R, Jones C, Ghiya N, Popovic T. CDC grand rounds: Prescription drug overdoses - A U.S. epidemic. Morbidity and Mortality Weekly Report. 2012;**61**(1):10-13

[14] Prunuske JP et al. Opioid prescribing patterns for non-malignant chronic pain for rural versus non-rural US adults: A population-based study using 2010 NAMCS data. BMC Health Services Research. 2014;**14**:563. DOI: 10.1186/s12913-014-0563-8

[15] US Center for Disease Control (CDC). 2018. Annual surveillance report of drug-related risks and outcomes. 2018. Available from: https://www.

drugabuse.gov/drugs-abuse/opioids/opioid-overdose-crisis

[16] Cicero TJ, Ellis MS, Surratt HL, Kurtz SP. The changing face of heroin use in the United States: A retrospective analysis of the past 50 years. JAMA Psychiatry. 2014;**71**(7):821-826. DOI: 10.1001/jamapsychiatry.2014.366

[17] Friedman J et al. Assessment of racial/ethnic and income disparities in the prescription of opioids and other controlled medications in California. JAMA Internal Medicine. 2019;**179**(4):469-476. DOI: 10.1001/jamainternmed.2018.6721

[18] Jones CM, Einstein EB, Compton WM. Changes in synthetic opioid involvement in drug overdose deaths in the United States, 2010-2016. JAMA. 2018;**319**(17):1819-1821. DOI: 10.1001/jama.2018.2844

[19] Berlin JA et al. Incidence of infective endocarditis in the delaware valley, 1988-1990. The American Journal of Cardiology. 1995;**76**(12):933-936

[20] Yew HS, Murdoch DR. Global trends in infective endocarditis epidemiology. Current Infectious Disease Reports. 2012;**14**(4):367-372. DOI: 10.1007/s11908-012-0265-5

[21] Sanaiha Y, Lyons R, Benharash P. Infective endocarditis in intravenous drug users. Trends in Cardiovascular Medicine. 2020;**30**(8):491-497. DOI: 10.1016/j.tcm.2019.11.007

[22] Slipczuk L et al. Infective endocarditis epidemiology over five decades: A systematic review. PLoS One. 2013;**8**(12):e82665. DOI: 10.1371/journal.pone.0082665

[23] Damlin A, Westling K. Patients with infective endocarditis and history of injection drug use in a Swedish referral hospital during 10 years. BMC Infectious Diseases. 2021;**21**(1):236. DOI: 10.1186/s12879-021-05914-1

[24] Murdoch DR et al. Clinical presentation, etiology, and outcome of infective endocarditis in the 21st century: The international collaboration on endocarditis-prospective cohort study. Archives of Internal Medicine. 2009;**169**(5):463-473. DOI: 10.1001/archinternmed.2008.603

[25] Bates MC, Annie F, Jha A, Kerns F. Increasing incidence of IV-drug use associated endocarditis in southern West Virginia and potential economic impact. Clinical Cardiology. 2019;**42**(4):432-437. DOI: 10.1002/clc.23162

[26] Leahey PA, LaSalvia MT, Rosenthal ES, Karchmer AW, Rowley CF. High morbidity and mortality among patients with sentinel admission for injection drug use-related infective endocarditis. Open Forum Infectious Diseases. 2019;**6**(4):ofz089. DOI: 10.1093/ofid/ofz089

[27] Kim JB et al. Surgical outcomes of infective endocarditis among intravenous drug users. The Journal of Thoracic and Cardiovascular Surgery. 2016;**152**(3):832-841.e1. DOI: 10.1016/j.jtcvs.2016.02.072

[28] Shmueli H, Thomas F, Flint N, Setia G, Janjic A, Siegel R. Right-sided infective endocarditis 2020: Challenges and updates in diagnosis and treatment. Journal of the American Heart Association. 2020;**9**(15):e017293. DOI: 10.1161/JAHA.120.017293

[29] Olsson RA, Romansky MJ. Staphylococcal tricuspid endocarditis in heroin addicts. Annals of Internal Medicine. 1962;**57**:755-762

[30] Cherubin CE, Neu HC. Infective endocarditis at the presbyterian hospital

in New York city from 1938-1967. The American Journal of Medicine. 1971;**51**(1):83-96

[31] Moss R, Munt B. Injection drug use and right sided endocarditis. Heart. 2003;**89**(5):577-581

[32] Chambers HF, Morris DL, Tauber MG, Modin G. Cocaine use and the risk for endocarditis in intravenous drug users. Annals of Internal Medicine. 1987;**106**(6):833-836

[33] Ortiz-Bautista C et al. Current profile of infective endocarditis in intravenous drug users: The prognostic relevance of the valves involved. International Journal of Cardiology. 2015;**187**:472-474. DOI: 10.1016/j.ijcard.2015.03.368

[34] Wilson LE, Thomas DL, Astemborski J, Freedman TL, Vlahov D. Prospective study of infective endocarditis among injection drug users. The Journal of Infectious Diseases. 2002;**185**(12):1761-1766. DOI: 10.1086/340827

[35] Thalme A, Westling K, Julander I. In-hospital and long-term mortality in infective endocarditis in injecting drug users compared to non-drug users: A retrospective study of 192 episodes. Scandinavian Journal of Infectious Diseases. 2007;**39**(3):197-204

[36] Heiro M et al. Infective endocarditis in a Finnish teaching hospital: A study on 326 episodes treated during 1980-2004. Heart. 2006;**92**(10):1457-1462. DOI: 10.1136/hrt.2005.084715

[37] Van der Meer J, Thompson J, Valkenburg H, Michel M. Epidemiology of bacterial endocarditis in The Netherlands. I. Patient characteristics. Archives of Internal Medicine. 1992;**152**(9). DOI: 10.1001/archinte.152.9.1863

[38] Gray ME, Rogawski McQuade ET, Scheld WM, Dillingham RA. Rising rates of injection drug use associated infective endocarditis in Virginia with missed opportunities for addiction treatment referral: A retrospective cohort study. BMC Infectious Diseases. 2018;**18**(1):532. DOI: 10.1186/s12879-018-3408-y

[39] Faber M, Frimodt-Moller N, Espersen F, Skinhoj P, Rosdahl V. Staphylococcus aureus endocarditis in Danish intravenous drug users: High proportion of left-sided endocarditis. Scandinavian Journal of Infectious Diseases. 1995;**27**(5):483-487

[40] Goyal A et al. Clinical characteristics and outcome of infective endocarditis among intravenous drug abusers in India. Indian Heart Journal. 2020;**72**(6):547-551. DOI: 10.1016/j.ihj.2020.09.014

[41] Graves MK, Soto L. Left-sided endocarditis in parenteral drug abusers: Recent experience at a large community hospital. Southern Medical Journal. 1992;**85**(4):378-380

[42] Mathew J, Addai T, Anand A, Morrobel A, Maheshwari P, Freels S. Clinical features, site of involvement, bacteriologic findings, and outcome of infective endocarditis in intravenous drug users. Archives of Internal Medicine. 1995;**155**(15):1641-1648

[43] Shrestha NK et al. Injection drug use and outcomes after surgical intervention for infective endocarditis. The Annals of Thoracic Surgery. 2015;**100**(3):875-882. DOI: 10.1016/j.athoracsur.2015.03.019

[44] Rabkin DG, Mokadam NA, Miller DW, Goetz RR, Verrier ED, Aldea GS. Long-term outcome for the surgical treatment of infective endocarditis with a focus on intravenous drug users. The Annals of Thoracic Surgery. 2012;**93**(1):51-57. DOI: 10.1016/j.athoracsur.2011.08.016

[45] Kaiser SP et al. Long-term outcomes in valve replacement surgery for infective endocarditis. The Annals of Thoracic Surgery. 2007;**83**(1):30-35. DOI: 10.1016/j.athoracsur.2006.07.037

[46] Hilbig A, Cheng A. Infective endocarditis in the intravenous drug use population at a tertiary hospital in Melbourne, Australia. Heart, Lung & Circulation. 2020;**29**(2). DOI: 10.1016/j.hlc.2018.12.016

[47] Carozza A et al. Infective endocarditis in intravenous drug abusers: Patterns of presentation and long-term outcomes of surgical treatment. The Journal of Heart Valve Disease. 2006;**15**(1):125-131

[48] Jain V, Yang MH, Kovacicova-Lezcano G, Juhle LS, Bolger AF, Winston LG. Infective endocarditis in an urban medical center: Association of individual drugs with valvular involvement. The Journal of Infection. 2008;**57**(2):132-138

[49] Peng S, French W, Pelikan P. Direct cocaine cardiotoxicity demonstrated by endomyocardial biopsy. Archives of Pathology & Laboratory Medicine. 1989;**113**(8):842-845

[50] Roux P, Carrieri MP, Keijzer L, Dasgupta N. Reducing harm from injecting pharmaceutical tablet or capsule material by injecting drug users. Drug and Alcohol Review. 2011;**30**(3):287-290

[51] Marchiori E, Lourenco S, Gasparetto TD, Zanetti G, Mano CM, Nobre LF. Pulmonary talcosis: Imaging findings. Lung. 2010;**188**(2):165-171. DOI: 10.1007/s00408-010-9230-y

[52] Keijzer L, Imbert E. The filter of choice: Filtration method preference among injecting drug users. Harm Reduction Journal. 2011;**8**:20

[53] Press P. Tampons, swabs and cigarette filters: The risky business of improvised filters. The Bulletin. 2018;**15**(2)

[54] Kerrigan SW, Clarke N, Loughman A, Meade G, Foster TJ, Cox D. Molecular basis for Staphylococcus aureus-mediated platelet aggregate formation under arterial shear in vitro. Arteriosclerosis, Thrombosis, and Vascular Biology. 2008;**28**(2):335-340. DOI: 10.1161/atvbaha.107.152058

[55] Herzberg MC. Platelet-streptococcal interactions in endocarditis. Critical Reviews in Oral Biology and Medicine. 1996;7(3):222-236

[56] Manning JE, Hume EB, Hunter N, Knox KW. An appraisal of the virulence factors associated with streptococcal endocarditis. Journal of Medical Microbiology. 1994;**40**(2):110-114. DOI: 10.1099/00222615-40-2-110

[57] Xiong YQ, Bensing BA, Bayer AS, Chambers HF, Sullam PM. Role of the serine-rich surface glycoprotein GspB of Streptococcus gordonii in the pathogenesis of infective endocarditis. Microbial Pathogenesis. 2008;**45**(4):297-301. DOI: 10.1016/j.micpath.2008.06.004

[58] Leask RL, Jain N, Butany J. Endothelium and valvular diseases of the heart. Microscopy Research and Technique. 2003;**60**(2):129-137. DOI: 10.1002/jemt.10251

[59] McCormick JK, Tripp TJ, Dunny GM, Schlievert PM. Formation of vegetations during infective endocarditis excludes binding of bacterial-specific host antibodies to Enterococcus faecalis. The Journal of Infectious Diseases. 2002;**185**(7):994-997. DOI: 10.1086/339604

[60] Durack DT, Beeson PB. Experimental bacterial endocarditis. II. Survival of

a bacteria in endocardial vegetations. British Journal of Experimental Pathology. 1972;**53**(1):50-53

[61] Frehel C, Hellio R, Cremieux AC, Contrepois A, Bouvet A. Nutritionally variant streptococci develop ultrastructural abnormalities during experimental endocarditis. Microbial Pathogenesis. 1988;**4**(4):247-255

[62] Baddour LM et al. Infective endocarditis in adults: Diagnosis, antimicrobial therapy, and management of complications: A scientific statement for healthcare professionals from the american heart association. Circulation. 2015;**132**(15):1435-1486. DOI: 10.1161/cir.0000000000000296

[63] Ye X et al. Right-sided infective endocarditis: The importance of vegetation size. Heart, Lung & Circulation. 2021 May;**30**(5):2021. DOI: 10.1016/j.hlc.2020.09.927

[64] Brink J, d'Udekem Y. So, vegetation size in right-sided endocarditis does not matter, or does it? Heart, Lung & Circulation. 2016;**25**(5):419-420. DOI: 10.1016/S1443-9506(16)30025-7

[65] Martin-Davila P et al. Analysis of mortality and risk factors associated with native valve endocarditis in drug users: The importance of vegetation size. American Heart Journal. 2005;**150**(5):1099-1106

[66] Habib G et al. ESC Guidelines for the management of infective endocarditis: The task force for the management of infective endocarditis of the european society of cardiology (ESC). Endorsed by: European association for cardio-thoracic surgery (EACTS), the European association of nuclear medicine (EANM). European Heart Journal. 2015, 2015;**36**(44):3075-3128. DOI: 10.1093/eurheartj/ehv319

[67] Kerridge BT et al. Gender and nonmedical prescription opioid use and DSM-5 nonmedical prescription opioid use disorder: Results from the National epidemiologic survey on alcohol and related conditions – III. Drug and Alcohol Dependence. 2015;**156**:47-56. DOI: 10.1016/j.drugalcdep.2015.08.026

[68] Marsh JC, Park K, Lin YA, Bersamira C. Gender differences in trends for heroin use and nonmedical prescription opioid use, 2007-2014. Journal of Substance Abuse Treatment. 2018;**87**:79-85. DOI: 10.1016/j.jsat.2018.01.001

[69] Green TC, Grimes Serrano JM, Licari A, Budman SH, Butler SF. Women who abuse prescription opioids: Findings from the addiction severity index-multimedia version connect prescription opioid database. Drug and Alcohol Dependence. 2009;**103**(1-2):65-73. DOI: 10.1016/j.drugalcdep.2009.03.014

[70] Back SE, Payne RL, Simpson AN, Brady KT. Gender and prescription opioids: Findings from the National survey on drug use and health. Addictive Behaviors. 2010;**35**(11):1001-1007. DOI: 10.1016/j.addbeh.2010.06.018

[71] Sung H-E, Tabachnick C, Feng L. Heroin injection among addicted felons: Testing extant theories. Deviant Behavior Interdisciplinary Journal. 2000;**21**:381-406

[72] Ross J et al. The characteristics of heroin users entering treatment: Findings from the Australian treatment outcome study (ATOS). Drug and Alcohol Review. 2005;**24**(5):411-418. DOI: 10.1080/09595230500286039

[73] Dwyer R, Richardson D, Ross MW, Wodak A, Miller ME, Gold J. A comparison of HIV risk between women and men who inject

drugs. AIDS Education and Prevention. 1994;**6**(5):379-389

[74] Spijkerman IJ, van Ameijden EJ, Mientjes GH, Coutinho RA, van den Hoek A. Human immunodeficiency virus infection and other risk factors for skin abscesses and endocarditis among injection drug users. Journal of Clinical Epidemiology. 1996;**49**(10):1149-1154

[75] Hope VD, Iversen J, Cullen KJ, Parry JV, Maher L, Nucbe F. Injection into the jugular vein among people who inject drugs in the United Kingdom: Prevalence, associated factors and harms. The International Journal on Drug Policy. 2017;**46**:28-33. DOI: 10.1016/j.drugpo.2017.05.005

[76] Bräu N, Esposito R, Simberkoff M. Cardiac valve replacement in patients infected with the human immunodeficiency virus. The Annals of Thoracic Surgery. 1992;**54**(3):552-554. DOI: 10.1016/0003-4975(92)90453-b

[77] Dominici C, Chello M. Impact of human immunodeficiency virus (HIV) infection in patients undergoing cardiac surgery: A systematic review. Reviews in Cardiovascular Medicine. 2020;**21**(3):411-418. DOI: 10.31083/j.rcm.2020.03.104

[78] Valencia Ortega M, Guinea J, Enrique A, Ortega G, Moreno V, González Lahoz J. Study of 42 cases of infective endocarditis in the HAART era in Spain. Clinical microbiology and Infection. The official publication of the European Society of Clinical Microbiology and Infectious Diseases. 2003;**9**(10):1073-1075. DOI: 10.1046/j.1469-0691.2003.00720.x

[79] Miro JM, del Rio A, Mestres CA. Infective endocarditis in intravenous drug abusers and HIV-1 infected patients. Infectious Disease Clinics of North America. 2002;**16**(2):273-295, vii-viii

[80] Bos J, Antonides C, Barth R, Klipstein-Grobusch K, Meel R, Vos A. Course of disease and clinical outcome of infective endocarditis in HIV-infected individuals: A systematic review and meta-analysis. AIDS Reviews. 2020;**22**(4):183-194. DOI: 10.24875/AIDSRev.19000117

[81] Pulvirenti JJ, Kerns E, Benson C, Lisowski J, Demarais P, Weinstein RA. Infective endocarditis in injection drug users: Importance of human immunodeficiency virus serostatus and degree of immunosuppression. Clinical Infectious Diseases. 1996;**22**(1):40-45. DOI: 10.1093/clinids/22.1.40

[82] Bassetti S, Battegay M. Staphylococcus aureus infections in injection drug users: Risk factors and prevention strategies. Infection. 2004;**32**(3):163-169

[83] Jackson KA et al. Invasive methicillin-resistant staphylococcus aureus infections among persons who inject drugs - Six sites, 2005-2016. Morbidity and Mortality Weekly Report. 2018;**67**(22):625-628. DOI: 10.15585/mmwr.mm6722a2

[84] Kluytmans J, van Belkum A, Verbrugh H. Nasal carriage of Staphylococcus aureus: Epidemiology, underlying mechanisms, and associated risks. Clinical Microbiology Reviews. 1997;**10**(3):505-520. DOI: 10.1128/CMR.10.3.505

[85] Tuazon C, Sheagren J. Increased rate of carriage of Staphylococcus aureus among narcotic addicts. The Journal of Infectious Diseases. 1974;**129**(6):725-727. DOI: 10.1093/infdis/129.6.725

[86] Lowy FD, Miller M. New methods to investigate infectious disease

transmission and pathogenesis--Staphylococcus aureus disease in drug users. The Lancet Infectious Diseases. 2002;**2**(10):605-612

[87] Asgeirsson H, Thalme A, Weiland O. Low mortality but increasing incidence of Staphylococcus aureus endocarditis in people who inject drugs: Experience from a Swedish referral hospital. Medicine. 2016;**95**(49):e5617. DOI: 10.1097/MD.0000000000005617

[88] Fowler VG Jr et al. Staphylococcus aureus endocarditis: A consequence of medical progress. JAMA. 2005;**293**(24):3012-3021. DOI: 10.1001/jama.293.24.3012

[89] Fowler VG Jr et al. Infective endocarditis due to Staphylococcus aureus: 59 prospectively identified cases with follow-up. Clinical Infectious Diseases. 1999;**28**(1):106-114

[90] Chambers HF, Korzeniowski OM, Sande MA. Staphylococcus aureus endocarditis: Clinical manifestations in addicts and nonaddicts. Medicine (Baltimore). 1983;**62**(3):170-177

[91] Miro JM, Moreno A, Mestres CA. Infective endocarditis in intravenous drug abusers. Current Infectious Disease Reports. 2003;**5**(4):307-316

[92] Garcia-Cabrera E et al. Neurological complications of infective endocarditis: Risk factors, outcome, and impact of cardiac surgery: A multicenter observational study. Circulation. 2013;**127**(23):2272-2284. DOI: 10.1161/circulationaha.112.000813

[93] Morelli M, Veve M, Lorson W, Shorman M. Candida spp. infective endocarditis: Characteristics and outcomes of twenty patients with a focus on injection drug use as a predisposing risk factor. Mycoses. 2021;**64**(2):181-186. DOI: 10.1111/myc.13200

[94] Badiee P, Amirghofran A, Ghazi Nour M, Shafa M, Nemati M. Incidence and outcome of documented fungal endocarditis. International Cardiovascular Research Journal. 2014;**8**(4):152-155

[95] Newton-John HF, Wise K, Looke DF. Role of the lemon in disseminated candidiasis of heroin abusers. The Medical Journal of Australia. 1984;**140**(13):780-781

[96] Bisbe J et al. Disseminated candidiasis in addicts who use brown heroin: Report of 83 cases and review. Clinical Infectious Diseases. 1992;**15**(6):910-923

[97] Albini T, Sun R, Holz E, Khurana R, Rao N. Lemon juice and Candida endophthalmitis in crack-cocaine misuse. The British Journal of Ophthalmology. 2007;**91**(5):702-703. DOI: 10.1136/bjo.2006.0108365

[98] Lankenau SE, Clatts MC, Goldsamt LA, Welle DL. Crack cocaine injection practices and HIV risk: Findings from New York and Bridgeport. Journal of Drug Issues. 2004;**34**(2):319-332

[99] Levine DP, Crane LR, Zervos MJ. Bacteremia in narcotic addicts at the Detroit Medical Center. II. Infectious endocarditis: A prospective comparative study. Reviews of Infectious Diseases. 1986;**8**(3):374-396

[100] Morpeth S et al. Non-HACEK gram-negative bacillus endocarditis. Annals of Internal Medicine. 2007;**147**(12):829-835

[101] Veve M, McCurry E, Cooksey G, Shorman M. Epidemiology and outcomes of non-HACEK infective endocarditis in the southeast United States. PLOS ONE.

2020;**15**(3):e0230199. DOI: 10.1371/journal.pone.0230199

[102] Loubet P et al. Endocarditis due to gram-negative bacilli at a French teaching hospital over a 6-year period: Clinical characteristics and outcome. Infectious Diseases. 2015;**47**(12). DOI: 10.3109/23744235.2015.1075660

[103] Bouza E, Muñoz P, Burillo A. Gram-negative endocarditis: Disease presentation, diagnosis and treatment. Current Opinion in Infectious Diseases. 2021;**34**(6). DOI: 10.1097/QCO.0000000000000788

[104] Rajashekaraiah K, Dhawan V, Rice T, McCulley D, Kallick C. Increasing incidence of Pseudomonas endocarditis among parenteral drug abusers. Drug and Alcohol Dependence. 1980;**6**(4). DOI: 10.1016/0376-8716(80)90327-0

[105] Reyes M, Ali A, Mendes R, Biedenbach D. Resurgence of Pseudomonas endocarditis in Detroit, 2006-2008. Medicine. 2009;**88**(5). DOI: 10.1097/MD.0b013e3181b8bedc

[106] McCann T, Elabd H, Blatt S, Brandt D. Intravenous drug use: A significant risk factor for Serratia Bacteremia. Therapeutic Advances in Infectious Disease. 2022;**9**:20499361221078116. DOI: 10.1177/20499361221078116

[107] Botsford KB, Weinstein RA, Nathan CR, Kabins SA. Selective survival in pentazocine and tripelennamine of Pseudomonas aeruginosa serotype O11 from drug addicts. The Journal of Infectious Diseases. 1985;**151**(2):209-216

[108] Kelly M, Yeager S, Shorman M, Wright L, Veve M. Incidence and predictors of gram-negative bacilli in hospitalized people who inject drugs with injection drug use-attributable infections. Antimicrobial Agents and Chemotherapy. 2021;**65**(12):e0092521. DOI: 10.1128/AAC.00925-21

[109] Tan C, Shojaei E, Wiener J, Shah M, Koivu S, Silverman M. Risk of new bloodstream infections and mortality among people who inject drugs with infective endocarditis. JAMA Network Open. 2020;**3**(8):e2012974. DOI: 10.1001/jamanetworkopen.2020.12974

[110] Baddour L, Meyer J, Henry B. Polymicrobial infective endocarditis in the 1980s. Reviews of Infectious Diseases. 1991;**13**(5):963-970. DOI: 10.1093/clinids/13.5.963

[111] Mehrzad R, Sublette M, Barza M. Polymicrobial endocarditis in intravenous heroin and fentanyl abuse. Journal of Clinical and Diagnostic Research. 2013;**7**(12):2981-2985. DOI: 10.7860/JCDR/2013/7303.3817

[112] Yuan SM. Mycobacterial endocarditis: A comprehensive review. Revista Brasileira de Cirurgia Cardiovascular. 2015;**30**(1):93-103. DOI: 10.5935/1678-9741.20140113

[113] Pérez-Jacoiste Asín M, Fernández-Ruiz M, Serrano-Navarro I, Prieto-Rodriguez S, Aguado J. Polymicrobial endocarditis involving Veillonella parvula in an intravenous drug user: Case report and literature review of Veillonella endocarditis. Infection. 2013;**41**(2):591-594. DOI: 10.1007/s15010-012-0398-3

[114] Jeurissen A, Stroy J, Wielenga R, Andriesse G. Severe infective endocarditis due to Neisseria sicca: Case report and review of literature. Acta Clinica Belgica. 2006;**61**(5):256-258. DOI: 10.1179/acb.2006.043

[115] Ho J, Archuleta S, Sulaiman Z, Fisher D. Safe and successful treatment of intravenous drug users with a peripherally

inserted central catheter in an outpatient parenteral antibiotic treatment service. The Journal of Antimicrobial Chemotherapy. 2010;**65**(12):2641-2644

[116] Rapoport AB, Fischer LS, Santibanez S, Beekmann SE, Polgreen PM, Rowley CF. Infectious diseases physicians' perspectives regarding injection drug use and related infections, United States, 2017. Open Forum Infectious Diseases. 2018;**5**(7):ofy132. DOI: 10.1093/ofid/ofy132

[117] Tookes H, Diaz C, Li H, Khalid R, Doblecki-Lewis S. A cost analysis of hospitalizations for infections related to injection drug use at a county safety-net hospital in Miami Florida. PLoS ONE. 2015;**10**(6):e0129360

[118] Yung D, Kottachchi D, Neupane B, Haider S, Loeb M. Antimicrobials for right-sided endocarditis in intravenous drug users: A systematic review. The Journal of Antimicrobial Chemotherapy. 2007;**60**(5):921-928. DOI: 10.1093/jac/dkm324

[119] Ribera E et al. Effectiveness of cloxacillin with and without gentamicin in short-term therapy for right-sided Staphylococcus aureus endocarditis. A randomized, controlled trial. Annals of Internal Medicine. 1996;**125**(12):969-974. DOI: 10.7326/0003-4819-125-12-199612150-00005

[120] Fortun J et al. Short-course therapy for right-side endocarditis due to Staphylococcus aureus in drug abusers: Cloxacillin versus glycopeptides in combination with gentamicin. Clinical Infectious Diseases. 2001;**33**(1):120-125

[121] Dworkin RJ, Lee BL, Sande MA, Chambers HF. Treatment of right-sided Staphylococcus aureus endocarditis in intravenous drug users with ciprofloxacin and rifampicin. Lancet. 1989;**2**(8671):1071-1073

[122] Cremieux AC et al. Evaluation of antibiotic diffusion into cardiac vegetations by quantitative autoradiography. The Journal of Infectious Diseases. 1989;**159**(5):938-944

[123] Robbins MJ, Frater RW, Soeiro R, Frishman WH, Strom JA. Influence of vegetation size on clinical outcome of right-sided infective endocarditis. The American Journal of Medicine. 1986;**80**(2):165-171

[124] Rohmann S et al. Prediction of rapid versus prolonged healing of infective endocarditis by monitoring vegetation size. Journal of the American Society of Echocardiography. 1991;**4**(5):465-474

[125] Gade ND, Qazi MS. Fluoroquinolone therapy in Staphylococcus aureus infections: Where Do We Stand? Journal of Lab Physicians. 2013;**5**(2):109-112

[126] Iversen K et al. Partial oral versus intravenous antibiotic treatment of endocarditis. The New England Journal of Medicine. 2019;**380**(5):415-424. DOI: 10.1056/NEJMoa1808312

[127] Spellberg B, Chambers H, Musher D, Walsh T, Bayer A. Evaluation of a paradigm shift from intravenous antibiotics to oral step-down therapy for the treatment of infective endocarditis: A narrative review. JAMA Internal Medicine. 2020;**180**(5):769-777. DOI: 10.1001/jamainternmed.2020.0555

[128] Meuris B et al. Durability of bioprosthetic aortic valves in patients under the age of 60 years - Rationale and design of the international INDURE registry. Journal of Cardiothoracic Surgery. 2020;**15**(1):119. DOI: 10.1186/s13019-020-01155-6

[129] Smyth BP, Barry J, Keenan E, Ducray K. Lapse and relapse following inpatient treatment of opiate dependence. Irish Medical Journal. 2010;**103**(6):176-179

[130] Cahill TJ, Prendergast BD. infective endocarditis. Lancet. 2016;**387**(10021):882-893. DOI: 10.1016/s0140-6736(15)00067-7

[131] An K et al. Infective endocarditis secondary to injection drug use: A survey of canadian cardiac surgeons. The Annals of Thoracic Surgery. 2021;**112**(5):1460-1467. DOI: 10.1016/j.athoracsur.2020.12.003

[132] DiMaio JM, Salerno TA, Bernstein R, Araujo K, Ricci M, Sade RM. Ethical obligation of surgeons to noncompliant patients: Can a surgeon refuse to operate on an intravenous drug-abusing patient with recurrent aortic valve prosthesis infection? The Annals of Thoracic Surgery. 2009;**88**(1):1-8. DOI: 10.1016/j.athoracsur.2009.03.088

[133] Hull SC, Jadbabaie F. When is enough enough? The dilemma of valve replacement in a recidivist intravenous drug user. The Annals of Thoracic Surgery. 2014;**97**(5):1486-1487. DOI: 10.1016/j.athoracsur.2014.02.010

[134] Mathew J, Abreo G, Namburi K, Narra L, Franklin C. Results of surgical treatment for infective endocarditis in intravenous drug users. Chest. 1995;**108**(1):73-77

[135] Pericàs J et al. Prospective cohort study of infective endocarditis in people who inject drugs. Journal of the American College of Cardiology. 2021;**77**(5). DOI: 10.1016/j.jacc.2020.11.062

[136] Bearpark L, Sartipy U, Franco-Cereceda A, Glaser N. Surgery for endocarditis in intravenous drug users. The Annals of Thoracic Surgery. 2021;**112**(2):573-581. DOI: 10.1016/j.athoracsur.2020.09.013

[137] Kilic A et al. Surgical treatment of infective endocarditis: Results in 831 patients from a single center. Journal of Cardiac Surgery. 2020;**35**(10):2725-2733. DOI: 10.1111/jocs.14893

[138] Witten J et al. Surgical treatment of right-sided infective endocarditis. The Journal of Thoracic and Cardiovascular Surgery. 2019;**157**(4):1418-1427.e14. DOI: 10.1016/j.jtcvs.2018.07.112

[139] Goodman-Meza D et al. Long term surgical outcomes for infective endocarditis in people who inject drugs: A systematic review and meta-analysis. BMC Infectious Diseases. 2019;**19**(1):918. DOI: 10.1186/s12879-019-4558-2

[140] Hall R et al. Drug use and postoperative mortality following valve surgery for infective endocarditis: A systematic review and meta-analysis. Clinical Infectious Diseases. 2019;**69**(7). DOI: 10.1093/cid/ciy1064

[141] Nguemeni Tiako MJ et al. Recidivism is the leading cause of death among intravenous drug users who underwent cardiac surgery for infective endocarditis. Seminars in Thoracic and Cardiovascular Surgery. 2019;**31**(1):40-45. DOI: 10.1053/j.semtcvs.2018.07.016

[142] Huang G, Barnes EW, Peacock JE Jr. Repeat infective endocarditis in persons who inject drugs: Take another little piece of my heart. Open Forum Infectious Diseases. 2018;**5**(12):ofy304. DOI: 10.1093/ofid/ofy304

[143] Alagna L et al. Repeat endocarditis: Analysis of risk factors based on the International collaboration on endocarditis - prospective cohort study. Clinical Microbiology and Infection. 2014;**20**(6):566-575. DOI: 10.1111/1469-0691.12395

[144] Klinker KP, Borgert SJ. Beyond vancomycin: The tail of the lipoglycopeptides. Clinical Therapeutics. 2015;**37**(12):2619-2636. DOI: 10.1016/j.clinthera.2015.11.007

[145] Madrigal AG, Basuino L, Chambers HF. Efficacy of Telavancin in a rabbit model of aortic valve endocarditis due to methicillin-resistant Staphylococcus aureus or vancomycin-intermediate Staphylococcus aureus. Antimicrobial Agents and Chemotherapy. 2005;**49**(8):3163-3165. DOI: 10.1128/aac.49.8.3163-3165.2005

[146] Nace H, Lorber B. Successful treatment of methicillin-resistant Staphylococcus aureus endocarditis with telavancin. The Journal of Antimicrobial Chemotherapy. 2010;**65**(6):1315-1316

[147] Joson J, Grover C, Downer C, Pujar T, Heidari A. Successful treatment of methicillin-resistant Staphylococcus aureus mitral valve endocarditis with sequential linezolid and telavancin monotherapy following daptomycin failure. The Journal of Antimicrobial Chemotherapy. 2011;**66**(9):2186-2188. DOI: 10.1093/jac/dkr234

[148] Marcos LA, Camins BC. Successful treatment of vancomycin-intermediate Staphylococcus aureus pacemaker lead infective endocarditis with telavancin. Antimicrobial Agents and Chemotherapy. 2010;**54**(12):5376-5378. DOI: 10.1128/aac.00857-10

[149] Lefort A, Pavie J, Garry L, Chau F, Fantin B. Activities of dalbavancin in vitro and in a rabbit model of experimental endocarditis due to Staphylococcus aureus with or without reduced susceptibility to vancomycin and teicoplanin. Antimicrobial Agents and Chemotherapy. 2004;**48**(3):1061-1064

[150] Steele JM, Seabury RW, Hale CM, Mogle BT. Unsuccessful treatment of methicillin-resistant Staphylococcus aureus endocarditis with dalbavancin. Journal of Clinical Pharmacy and Therapeutics. 2018;**43**(1):101-103. DOI: 10.1111/jcpt.12580

[151] Tobudic S et al. Dalbavancin as primary and sequential treatment for Gram-positive infective endocarditis: 2-Year experience at the general hospital of Vienna. Clinical Infectious Diseases. 2018;**67**(5):795-798. DOI: 10.1093/cid/ciy279

[152] Saleh-Mghir A et al. Activity and diffusion of LY333328 in experimental endocarditis due to vancomycin-resistant Enterococcus faecalis. Antimicrobial Agents and Chemotherapy. 1999;**43**(1):115-120

[153] Wunsch S et al. Multicenter clinical experience of real life Dalbavancin use in gram-positive infections. International Journal of Infectious Diseases. 2019;**81**:210-214. DOI: 10.1016/j.ijid.2019.02.013

[154] Bryson-Cahn C et al. Dalbavancin as secondary therapy for serious staphylococcus aureus infections in a vulnerable patient population. Open Forum Infectious Diseases. 2019;**6**(2):ofz028. DOI: 10.1093/ofid/ofz028

[155] Pfaller MA, Sader HS, Rhomberg PR, Flamm RK. In vitro activity of delafloxacin against contemporary bacterial pathogens from the United States and Europe. Antimicrobial Agents and Chemotherapy. 2014;**61**(4):2017. DOI: 10.1128/aac.02609-16

[156] Jorgensen SCJ, Mercuro NJ, Davis SL, Rybak MJ. Delafloxacin: Place in therapy and review of microbiologic, clinical and pharmacologic properties. Infectious Disease and Therapy. 2018;**7**(2):197-217. DOI: 10.1007/s40121-018-0198-x

[157] Aranaga C, Pantoja L, Martínez E, Falco A. Phage therapy in the era of multidrug resistance in bacteria: A systematic review. International Journal

of Molecular Sciences. 2022;**23**(9):4577. DOI: 10.3390/ijms23094577

[158] Suh G et al. Considerations for the use of phage therapy in clinical practice. Antimicrobial Agents and Chemotherapy. 2022;**66**(3):e0207121. DOI: 10.1128/AAC.02071-21

[159] Oechslin F et al. Synergistic interaction between phage therapy and antibiotics clears pseudomonas aeruginosa infection in endocarditis and reduces virulence. The Journal of Infectious Diseases. 2017;**215**(5):703-712. DOI: 10.1093/infdis/jiw632

[160] Gilbey T, Ho J, Cooley L, Petrovic Fabijan A, Iredell J. Adjunctive bacteriophage therapy for prosthetic valve endocarditis due to Staphylococcus aureus. The Medical Journal of Australia. 2019;**211**(3):142-143.e1. DOI: 10.5694/mja2.50274

[161] Petrovic Fabijan A, Lin R, Ho J, Maddocks S, Ben Zakour N, Iredell J. Safety of bacteriophage therapy in severe Staphylococcus aureus infection. Nature Microbiology. 2020;**5**(3):465-472. DOI: 10.1038/s41564-019-0634-z

[162] Abubakar H, Rashed A, Subahi A, Yassin A, Shokr M, Elder M. AngioVac system used for vegetation debulking in a patient with tricuspid valve endocarditis: A case report and review of the literature. Case Reports in Cardiology. 2017;**2017**:1923505. DOI: 10.1155/2017/1923505

[163] Enezate T, Alkhatib D, Raja J, Chinta V, Patel M, Omran J. AngioVac for minimally invasive removal of intravascular and intracardiac masses: A systematic review. Current Cardiology Reports. 2022;**24**(4):377-382. DOI: 10.1007/s11886-022-01658-9

[164] Rosenthal ES, Karchmer AW, Theisen-Toupal J, Castillo RA, Rowley CF. Suboptimal addiction interventions for patients hospitalized with injection drug use-associated infective endocarditis. The American Journal of Medicine. 2016;**129**(5):481-485. DOI: 10.1016/j.amjmed.2015.09.024

[165] Simon R, Snow R, Wakeman S. Understanding why patients with substance use disorders leave the hospital against medical advice: A qualitative study. Substance Abuse. 2020;**41**(4):519-525. DOI: 10.1080/08897077.2019.1671942

[166] Liebschutz JM et al. Buprenorphine treatment for hospitalized, opioid-dependent patients: A randomized clinical trial. JAMA Internal Medicine. 2014;**174**(8):1369-1376. DOI: 10.1001/jamainternmed.2014.2556

[167] Cushman PA, Liebschutz JM, Anderson BJ, Moreau MR, Stein MD. Buprenorphine initiation and linkage to outpatient buprenorphine do not reduce frequency of injection opiate use following hospitalization. Journal of Substance Abuse Treatment. 2016;**68**:68-73. DOI: 10.1016/j.jsat.2016.06.003

[168] Islam S et al. Reducing injection intensity is associated with decreased risk for invasive bacterial infection among high-frequency injection drug users. Harm Reduction Journal. 2019;**16**(1):38. DOI: 10.1186/s12954-019-0312-8

Chapter 5

Infective Endocarditis in Congenital Heart Disease

Naomi Nakagawa

Abstract

Any congenital heart disease (CHD) with high-velocity jets of blood flow and/or artificial material is associated with the highest risk of infective endocarditis (IE). And IE can be a big issue not only for the patient with CHD before the operation but also after the palliative and the radical surgery. Jets stream of the intracardiac shunt (including the residual shunt after corrective operation) and artificial conduits and/or patches after palliated or corrective operation can be the origin of IE. Even though the incidence of IE in children is much lower than in adults, the risk of IE can be high for patients with CHD. Certain CHD are common underlying conditions of IE, including ventricular septal defects, patent ductus arteriosus, aortic valve abnormalities, endocardial cushion defects, and tetralogy of Fallot. Furthermore, patients with complex cyanotic CHD with or without conduit procedures, palliative shunt, patches, and prosthetic valves are becoming a large group at risk.

Keywords: congenital heart disease, artificial material, high-velocity jet, cyanotic congenital heart disease, palliative operation

1. Introduction

Many of congenital heart diseases (CHD) have become manageable because of the progress of medical and surgical approaches and the improvement of prosthetic materials over the past few decades. Infective endocarditis (IE) can be a big issue not only for the patient after the radical surgery but also after the palliative surgery and before any operation. Because most of them have a condition that can predispose them to IE, including valve regurgitation, jet flow of intra/extracardiac shunt, and prosthetic material. Even though the number of cases of IE in children is small compared to adults, recent reports have pointed out a tendency that the incidence of IE among children is increasing due to the improving survival rate of patients with CHD [1–3] and more frequent use of implanted prosthetic material [4–7].

2. Epidemiology

Now CHD appears to be the predominant underlying condition for IE, especially in children over 2 years old [2, 4] and age of IE gets younger because of early advanced treatment [8, 9]. Pediatric IE related to CHD accounts for 74–88% of the total pediatric IE [10, 11]. Age distribution seems with a peak in infancy during childhood [1, 8, 11, 12].

In children with CHD, the cumulative incidence of IE has been estimated at 6.1 per 1000 patients, and overall incidence rates of IE are 4.1 to 11.13 per 10,000 person-years [8, 13, 14]. And children with CHD have an estimated 15–140 times higher risk of developing IE compared to the general population [10]. The lesion group-specific cumulative incidence of IE was reported as follows: cyanotic CHD, 31.0–35.73; atrioventricular septal defect, 11.1–27.24; left-sided lesions (e.g., coarctation of the aorta, aortic stenosis/insufficiency, mitral stenosis/insufficiency), 7.9–14.3; ventricular septal defect, 3.2–10.1; right sided-lesion (e.g., Ebstein's anomaly, tricuspid valve disease, anomalous of pulmonary valve/artery), 3.0–4.2; atrial septal defect, 2.8–3.0; and patent ductus arteriosus, 1.5–3.2 [8, 13].

IE is a serious problem not only for pediatric CHD but also the adult CHD. An increasing number of children reach adulthood because of the improvement in medical and surgical procedures. The number of adult CHD patients is now exceeding number of children with CHD, and they are the much more vulnerable to IE due to greater cardiac complexity and higher rates of comorbidities compared to a few decades ago [3]. The overall incidence of endocarditis in adults with CHD has been reported to be 11 per 100 000 person-years, and this incidence is three times higher than in children with CHD [15] and which is a considerable increase compared with the general population, in which a rate of 1.5 to 6.0 per 100 000 patient-years [15, 16]. In general, IE is correlated with age, and patients with CHD have a similar IE incidence as that of 81-year-old control. But by the age of 40–65 years, the IE incidence is more than 75–100 times higher in patients with CHD than in controls [17, 18]. And the risk of adult CHD was 2.5 times higher in children with CHD [18].

Overall inpatient mortality of IE in patients with CHD is estimated at 5.0–6.7% in children [1, 13] and up to 8.8–15% in adults [14, 18], and mortality of IE patients with cyanotic CHD is 3.6 times higher than that of the IE patients with non-cyanotic CHD [13]. Mortality rate is up to 48% in patients with tetralogy of Fallot and pulmonary atresia and 9.9% in patients of tetralogy of Fallot without pulmonary atresia.

3. Risk factors

All vegetations occur in areas where there is a pressure gradient with resulting turbulence blood flow [3]. Congenital heart disease with high- velocity jets of blood flow and/or artificial material is associated with the highest risk of IE. Any lesion associated with turbulence of blood flow, with or without shunting, can be a basement for IE [2]. Certain CHD are still common underlying conditions of IE, including ventricular septal defects, patent ductus arteriosus, aortic valve abnormalities, endocardial cushion defects, and tetralogy of Fallot [8, 19, 20]. Furthermore, patients with complex cyanotic CHD with or without conduit procedures, palliative shunt, patches, and prosthetic valves are becoming the large group at risk [2], even though mechanisms of cyanosis on the pathogenesis of IE are not clear [9]. On the other hand, in secundum atrial septal defect which has no high-velocity jet flow shunting, and in mild pulmonic stenosis, endocarditis is not likely to occur [2, 20].

Turbulent blood flow from a high-to low-pressure chamber or across a narrowed orifice traumatizes the endothelium. Thrombogenesis can occur on the damaged endothelium easily and results in the disposition of sterile clumps of platelets and fibrin and the formation of nonbacterial thrombotic endocarditis [3]. This provides an environment to which bacteria can adhere and eventually form infected vegetation. This endothelial lesion is usually located at the low-pressure end of an abnormality with a large gradient and most vegetations are found on the atrial side of the atrioventricular valves and downstream in the descending aorta in coarctation of the aorta [3, 21]. An exception is valvular aortic stenosis. The vegetation occurs often on the ventricular side of the aortic valve. A possible explanation is that almost all aortic valvular stenosis is accompanied by some degree of aortic insufficiency [3]. And an aortic regurgitant jet or prolapsing aortic vegetation can affect the anterior mitral leaflet causing secondary vegetation [21].

Approximately 50–70% of IE in children with CHD have had previous cardiac surgery, particularly palliative shunt, or complex corrective surgery [3, 4, 13]. Prosthetic material with higher surface tension (e.g., polyethylene, terephthalate) exhibits higher binding capacity for fibrinogen, a hydrated macromolecule, than material with lower surface tension (e.g., fluorocarbon polymers) and is more prone to initiate IE [9]. Even though complete repair of CHD with sufficient endothelialization after 6 months of procedure may eliminate the risk for IE, patients are at high risk before complete endothelialization. Patients who had undergone cardiac surgery in the prior 6 months are more than 5 times more likely to develop IE compared to patients without cardiac surgery [8, 13]. Among the invasive procedure, shunt surgery is associated higher risk of developing IE within the 6 months after procedure [13]. In addition, postoperative IE is a long-term risk even after corrective surgery, especially in those with residual defects, surgical shunt, and other prosthetic material [4, 9].

The progress of transcatheter placement of devices such as septal or vascular occluders, vascular occluders, and coils can be another risk factor for IE. Generally, IE occurs particularly in the early post-deployment period before endothelialization especially within 6 months [4, 13], and it is rare to occur after complete endothelialization. And it is suggested that IE after transcatheter device treatment is related to residual defects or shunts after device deployment [22].

Pulmonary valve implantation is often required in patients with CHD, and transcatheter pulmonary valve implantation is increasingly being used. Multiple studies which analyzed the occurrence of IE in surgically and transcatheter implanted bovine jugular vein pulmonary conduits, such as Melody valve stents and Contegra conduits, reported an increased incidence of IE compared to other valve types [23–25]. Annualized incidence rates of IE in homografts, Contegra and Melody valves were 0.40%, 0.97%, and 6.96% 1 year and 0.27%, 1.12%, and 2.89% 5 years after valve implantation [24]. And a systematic review reported that the median cumulative incidence of IE was higher for bovine jugular vein valve compared with other valves (5.4% vs. 1.2%) and the incidence of IE was not different between surgical and catheter-based valve implantation. They concluded that this result suggested that the substrate for future infection is related to the tissue rather than the method of implantation [25].

Several predictors for IE in adult CHD patients are identified. Foremost among these predictors are recent (<6 months) medical interventions including genitourinary, gastrointestinal, and respiratory procedures (Odds Ratio 12.52), recent (<6 months) cardiac surgery (OR 9.07), male sex (OR 2.07), and diabetes mellitus (OR 1.65) [18]. And previous IE is a substantial risk factor of recurrent IE [9]. Regarding CHD lesions, endocardial cushion defect (OR 6.65) and left-sided lesions (including aortic coarctation, aortic stenosis/insufficiency, mitral stenosis/insufficiency) (OR 5.11), cyanotic CHD (OR 4.82), and ventricular septal defect (OR 2.81) are at higher IE risk. Because ventricular septal defect is the most frequent CHD, it can be the most frequent CHD-associated IE if unrepaired [9]. And right-sided lesions (including Ebstein's disease, anomalous pulmonary artery/valve, and tricuspid valve disease), atrial septal defects, and patent ductus arteriosus are at lowest IE risk [18]. Patients palliated by an aortopulmonary shunt, such as Glenn anastomosis and Fontan procedure can survive until adulthood recently and can be predicted to increasingly contribute to further numbers of IE [9].

4. Clinical findings

Pediatric IE presents non-specific symptoms and it creates a diagnostic challenge for clinicians and this is one of the reasons that high mortality of pediatric IE due to the failure to effectively- recognized it [10]. The most frequent symptoms and clinical signs are the same as IE without CHD, fever (>80%), malaise, fatigue, weight loss, arthralgia, headache, chills, and myalgia. Valvular lesions that produce leaflet destruction result in regurgitant murmurs, in contrast, the change of the heart murmur may not be recognizable in CHD with high-velocity jet flow shunting. Congestive heart failure occurs in up to half of the IE in CHD patients and is the leading cause of hemodynamic compromise due to the destruction of affected valves [9]. The frequency of cardiac episode-related complications in IE with CHD is equivalent to adults with structural heart disease [9]. In patients with cyanotic CHD and who have undergone systemic-pulmonary artery shunt, diminution of a continuous murmur and declining systemic oxygen saturation may reflect graft infection with obstruction of blood flow [2–4]. The endocarditis of patent ductus arteriosus or coarctation of the aorta can cause aneurysm formation and may rupture [21].

Even though Roth's spots, Janeway lesions, Osler nodes, petechiae, Splinter hemorrhages, and splenomegaly are considerably less common in children compared to adults IE [2–4, 10], extracardiac episode-related complications of IE in CHD are frequent (up to 43%) and either caused by embolic events or immune phenomena [9]. Extracardiac manifestations of IE including emboli to the abdominal vessels, brain, and coronary arteries may produce severe symptoms associated with ischemia and/or hemorrhage [2]. Although systemic emboli by bacterial vegetation in the right heart rarely occurs because of filtration by the lungs [3], it can occur when the patient has right to left shunt such as cyanotic CHD (**Figure 1**) [21]. Although it is not frequent, pulmonary valve involvement can be seen more often in patients with in CHD than patients without CHD (**Figure 2**) [7]. Right-sided IE can cause chest pain, pulmonary infarction, pneumonitis, abscess, or asthma-like symptoms related to septic pulmonary embolization (**Figure 3**) [7, 21]. Chest X-ray shows infiltrative shadow when emboli to pulmonary arterial branches, and lung perfusion scintigraphy can indicate the lack of blood perfusion of this area (**Figure 4**) helps to differentiate from simple pneumonia.

Considering the results from many reports, vegetation size and location have a strong influence on the extracardiac episode-related complications and mortality [11, 26–28]. A vegetation size of ≥10 mm for left-sided IE and 20 mm for right-sided IE in adult patients is associated with a higher mortality [27–30]. Especially for infants or small children, it seems to be more suitable to take into vegetation size relative to patient body size [11, 28]. Vegetation size adjusted for body surface area was a significant independent predictor of early mortality and overall mortality for left-sided IE in

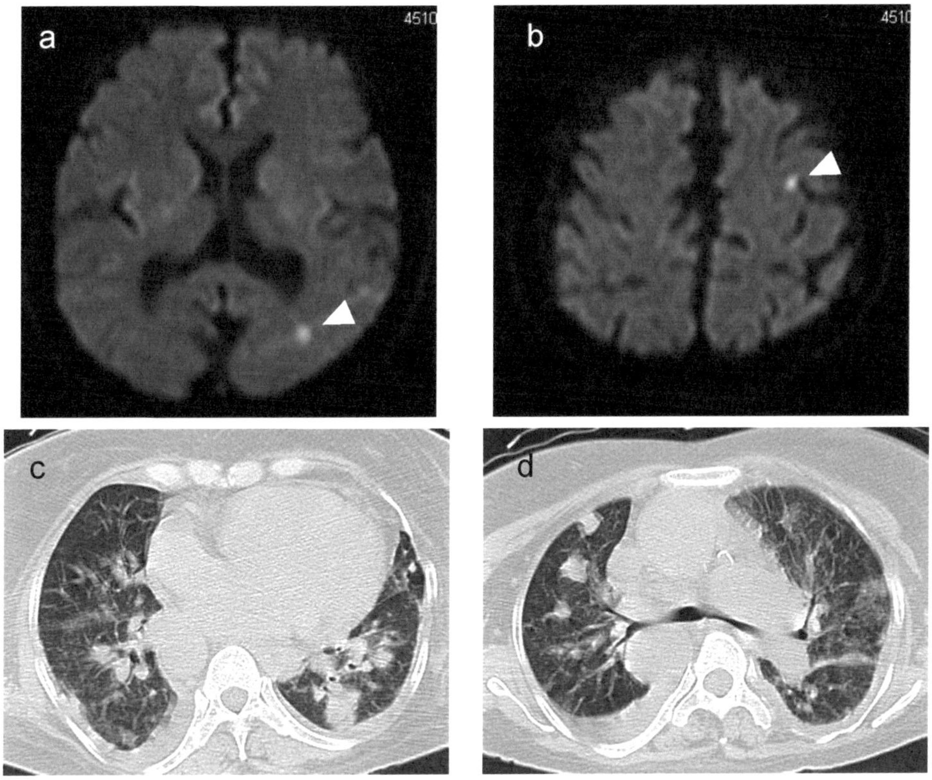

Figure 1.
Brain CT findings of brain emboli by bacterial vegetation in the right heart in a patient with right to left shunt (a, b). Vegetations were detected on the tricuspid valve of a patient with unrepaired single ventricle physiology and many bacterial emboli in the lung were detected by chest CT at the same time (c, d).

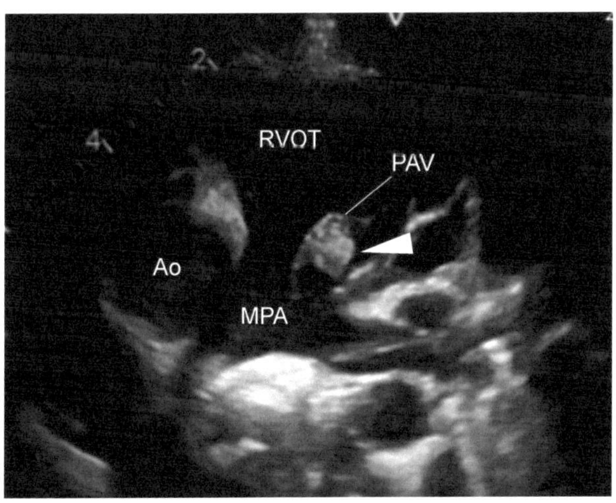

Figure 2.
Transthoracic short axis echocardiogram in a patient with ventricular septal defect and two chambered right ventricle. Bacterial vegetation adhered to pulmonary valve (white triangle). Ao: Aorta, MPA: main pulmonary artery, PAV: pulmonary arteria valve, RVOT: right ventricle outlet tract.

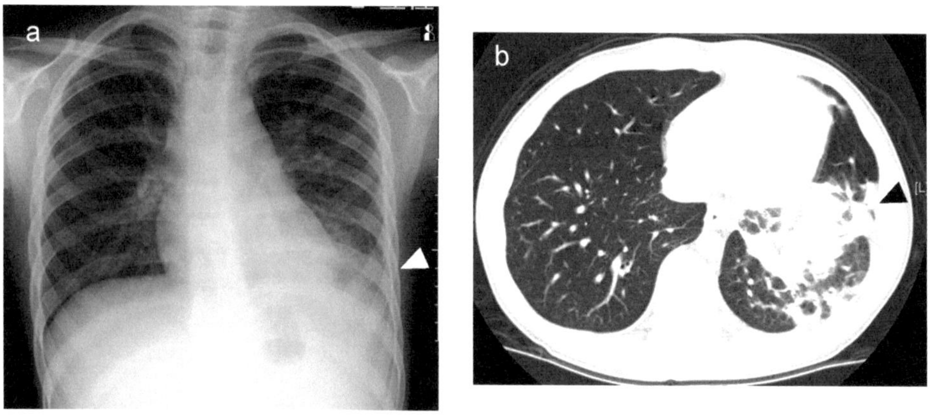

Figure 3.
Septic pulmonary embolization and pneumonitis in a patient with unrepaired ventricular septal defect. Original bacterial vegetation was detected on the pulmonary valve. It disappeared when the patient complained of severe chest pain and chest X-ray finding showed infiltration.

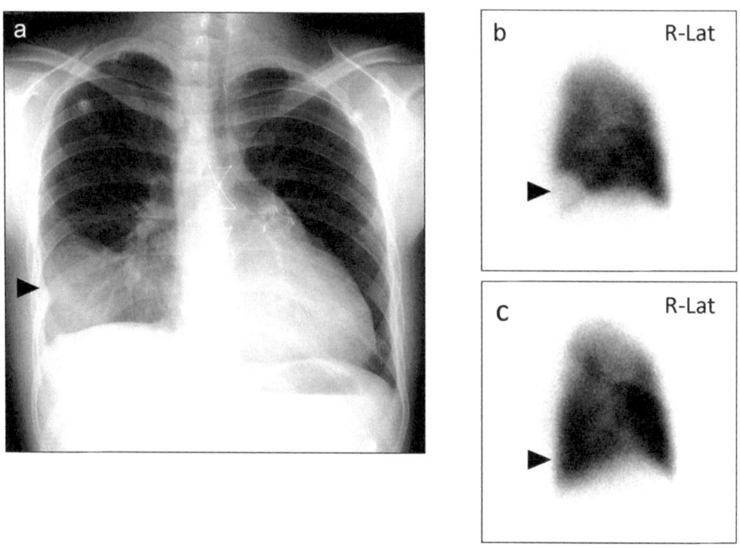

Figure 4.
Emboli to pulmonary arterial branches in a patient with Truncus arteriosus repaired by Rastelli procedure. Chest X-ray showed infiltrative shadow (a) and lung perfusion scintigraphy indicated the luck of blood perfusion of this area (b). The photo of 2 years before showed no lack of perfusion in the same area (c).

children and absolute vegetation size was not correlated with any adverse events [11]. The relative risk of operative mortality increased by 7% for every 1 mm/m^2 increase in vegetation size, and the absolute risk of operative mortality increased by 1.1% [11].

5. Microbiology

Blood culture should be indicated for all patients with CHD and/or previous cardiac endocarditis when patients have fever of unexplained origin. It is important to obtain adequate volumes of blood from patients including children and infants.

But it is difficult and unfeasible to obtain the large amounts which are recommended for adults. Lesser amounts are optimal [4], for example, 1 to 3 ml in infants and young children and 5 to 7 ml in older children [2]. Three blood cultures should be obtained separately from different venipuncture sites on the first day, and two more blood cultures are recommended if there is no growth by the second day of incubation [2, 4]. Three separate blood cultures from venipuncture sites can be undergone over a brief period and empiric therapy is started because therapy should not be delayed in patients with acute IE [2–4]. If all the blood culture is negative, antibiotics can be withheld for >48 hours until further blood cultures are obtained when the patients are not severely ill and are clinically stable without signs of altered mental status or hemodynamic compromise [4]. Taking a blood culture of arterial blood is not recommended because it is not more useful than venipuncture. It does not increase yield over venous blood cultures [4].

Most frequently isolated organisms in IE patients with CHD are Gram-positive cocci, including Viridans group streptococci (VGS: e.g., Streptococcus sanguis, S mitis group, S mutans), staphylococci (both S aureus and coagulase-negative staphylococci (CoNS)), β-hemolytic streptococci, and enterococci [2]. Among them, Viridans group streptococci (VGS) are generally the most frequently isolated organisms [4, 9]. Staphylococcus aureus is usually the second most common cause of IE but the increasing percentage of Staphylococcus aureus-related IE is pointed out [3] and is now the most common cause in some studies [11] and is the most common agent of rapidly progressive IE [4]. Coagulase-negative staphylococci (CoNS) is the third most common bacterial isolate [11] and is seen more commonly in patients with prosthetic valves compared to native valves [9, 11]. The difference in the frequency of CoNS infection in pediatric CHD between prosthetic valve IE and native valve IE is approximately three times [11]. And this relationship is in accord with reports of IE in adult CHD [31]. Enterococcal endocarditis is relatively less common in children than in adults. Less frequently, other organisms such as the HACEK group of organisms (HACEK: Haemophilus species, Aggregatibacter species, Cardiobacterium hominis, Eikenella corrodens, and Kingella species) are implicated [2, 9].

In infants, IE caused by Streptococcal viridans is rare and most cases caused by CoNS, fungi, or Staphylococcus aureus [8, 20].

IE associated with implanted prosthetic material frequently is caused by Staphylococcus aureus or CoNS. These organisms often are implanted at the time of surgery, and infection manifests within 60 days after cardiac surgery, but CoNS infection may present as late as ≥1 year after surgery [3, 4].

Culture-negative IE is not neglectable problem for patients with CHD. The prevalence of culture-negative IE is 5–12% [2, 3, 9]. The most common cause of culture-negative IE is current/recent antibiotic therapy or infection caused by a fastidious organism that grows poorly in vitro [9, 21]. And withdrawing of antibiotics for >48 hours should be considered to obtain further blood cultures when the patients are not severely ill [4].

6. Diagnostic imaging

Echocardiography is mandatory on any patient with suspicious of IE. In most pediatric cases, transthoracic echocardiography (TTE) is adequate for initial examination [32] because high-quality images can generally be obtained compared to adults and TTE is more sensitive in the pediatric patients than in adult patients for detection of vegetation [2]. And in young children and infants, transesophageal echocardiography (TEE) can be difficult to be undergone without general anesthesia. TEE should be considered if transthoracic windows are poor with difficulty to gain the complete visualization of higher-risk structures because of a prominent lung artifact, prosthetic valve, or material that is positioned behind the sternum or other location not well-visualized by transthoracic images [2–4, 32]. TEE should be undergone without delay if the IE was highly suspected and abnormal findings were not detected by transthoracic echocardiography [32]. The absence of vegetations on echocardiography does not deny the presence of IE including the finding by TEE [2, 33]. There is a very important consideration in patients with both of repaired and unrepaired CHD, who can have vegetations located in areas not readily visible even though by TEE (e.g., Blalock-Taussig shunt) [2, 33]. And it is revealed that IE among the patients with CHD are less likely to have visible vegetations irrespective of whether TTE or TEE is used [21]. On the other hand, echogenic masses can represent a sterile thrombus, sterile prosthetic materials, or normal anatomic variation rather than an infected vegetation [2].

When diagnosing endomyocardial damage using echocardiography is challenging especially in patients with prosthetic materials, cardiac computed tomography (CT) is a significant alternative method for diagnosis of IE [34]. Cardiac CT functions at a high specificity in IE of prosthetic valve and other prosthetic materials including shunts and conduits [35]. Cardiac CT is also useful to identify extra-cardiac features related to IE such as septic emboli (**Figure 5**) [36].

18F-fluorodeoxyglucose positron emission tomography/CT (18F-FDG PET/CT) is a molecular functional imaging technique and an emerging technology being used to diagnose endomyocardial damage. 18F-FDG PET/CT detects inflammation in the heart, especially around prosthetic materials and systemic inflammatory lesions caused by septic embolisms [10, 34, 37]. Although the diagnostic capability of 18F-FDG PET/CT is limited by low sensitivity in patients with native valve endocarditis probably due to its low sensitivity for detecting highly mobile small vegetations, 18F-FDG PET/CT is useful for diagnosing prosthetic valve endocarditis and perivalvular abscesses not only in left-sided IE but also in right-sided IE. Therefore, in patients with CHD and prosthetic materials and who are clinically suspected of IE, 18F-FDG PET/CT may be incorporated in the initial workup to increase the diagnostic sensitivity [34, 37].

7. Treatment

In general, the strategy of treatment of IE associated with CHD is comparable to that with IE not associated with CHD and antibiotic therapy is the mainstay of therapy. Guidelines for antibiotic therapy of IE have been published by the American Heart Association (AHA) and the European Society of Cardiology (ESC) [38, 39]. A prolonged course of therapy (at least 2 weeks and often 4 to 8 weeks) is necessary because infecting organisms are embedded within the fibrin-platelet matrix and exist in remarkably high concentrations with relatively low rates of bacterial metabolism and cell division, which results in decreased susceptibility of β-lactam and other cell wall-active antibiotics [2, 3, 9]. And cure of IE requires sterilizing vegetations [3, 9]. Bactericidal rather than bacteriostatic antibiotics must be administrated in high dosages whenever possible to decrease the possibility of treatment failures or relapses

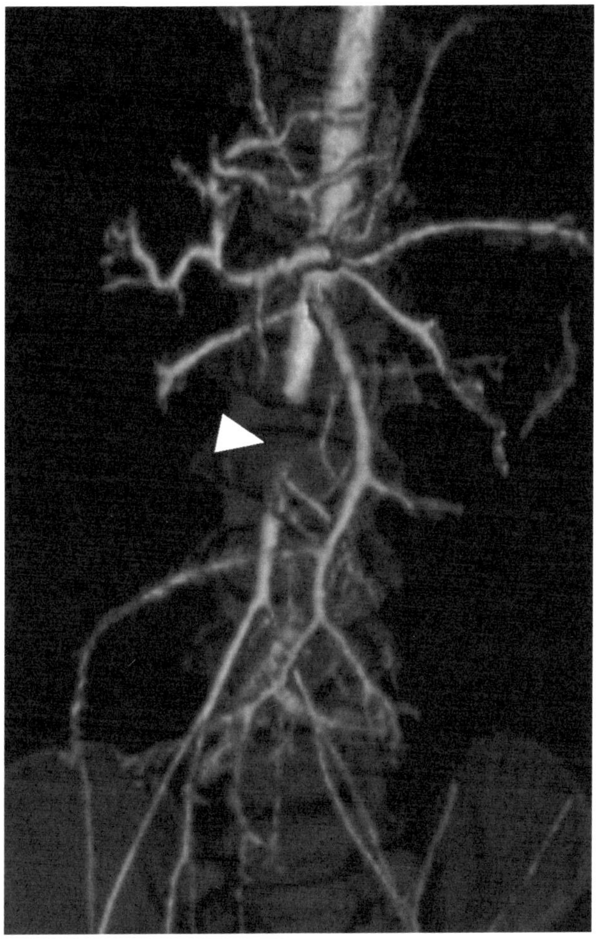

Figure 5.
Emboli of abdominal aorta by infective vegetation in a patient with tetralogy of Fallot with pulmonary atresia (white triangle). Poor blood circulation on the lower extremities was detected, and CT findings revealed obstructed descending aorta. Original fungal vegetation was located on the right atrium.

of IE [2, 3, 9]. Intravenous therapy is much preferable to oral to achieve higher serum antibiotics level. The course of antibiotic therapy varies based on the pathogen and the sites involved in the primary infection and any potential embolic sites [32]. Prosthetic material related IE and Staphylococcal IE are well known as complicated condition and recommended to be treated for longer period at least 4 to 6 weeks. Bacteremia generally resolves within several days after initiation of the appropriate antibiotics with enough dosages [2, 9]. 75% of patients become afebrile during first week and 95% during second week of appropriate antibiotic therapy. Work up to detect pathogen must be repeated when fever persists beyond this period, even though drug fever as a side effect of antibiotics must be considered [9]. Blood cultures should be performed at the end of the treatment and 4 weeks after completion of antibiotic therapy to check the relapse of infection [3, 9].

Fungal IE remains difficult to treat and mortality is up to 20 to 50% [3]. Even after combined intravenous antifungal management and surgical therapy, an on-going long-term antifungal therapy is often necessary to prevent a relapse of IE [9].

8. Surgery

Cardiac surgery is performed in approximately 16–20% of in IE patients with CHD [1, 9]. The three main indications of early surgery for IE are heart failure, prevention of embolic events and uncontrolled infection [39]. But the ideal timing for surgery is controversial subject in both of pediatric and adult IE related to CHD [9]. There is no indication of the surgical management only for IE in CHD patients and it is an extension of guideline for usual adult IE patients [4]. Surgery is considered for IE related to CHD with persistent bacteremia despite antimicrobial treatments, large mobile vegetations, prosthetic valves, prolonged clinical symptoms lasting more than 3 months, myocardial abscess formation with suspicions of atrioventricular block, mycotic aneurysms (**Figure 6**), previous IE, Staphylococcus aureus IE, left-sided IE, presence of systemic-to-pulmonary shunts, cyanotic CHD, and fungal IE [3, 4, 9]. The preventive operation for primary embolic events remains controversial because conflicting data on potential predictor of embolization were shown [26, 40]. Prediction of the embolic events remains difficult even in the adult IE [39]. An 'embolic risk calculator' were created to assess the embolic risk and evaluate the necessity of a surgery using six factors (age, diabetes, atrial fibrillation, previous embolism, vegetation length, and S. aureus infection) which associated with increased risk [41], but it is not suitable for pediatric patients. The highest risk of new embolism is seen during the first 2 weeks, especially first few days following initiation of antibiotic therapy and the risk rapidly decreases [42, 43]. For this reason, the benefit of surgery to prevent embolic events are greatest during the first 2 weeks of antibiotic therapy [39].

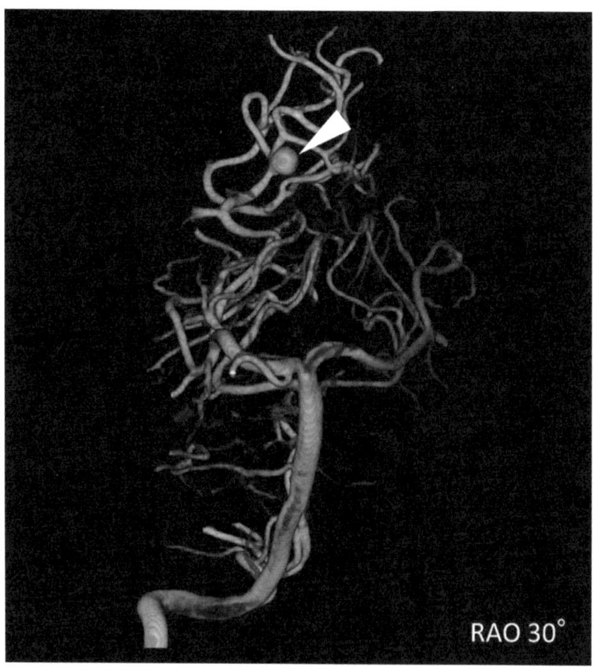

Figure 6.
A mycotic aneurysm in a patient with repaired tetralogy of Fallot (white triangle). A vegetation was detected on the mitral valve.

The overall operative mortality is reported as 5.8–15% in pediatric IE and 16.4% among adults [11, 12, 44]. Younger age, prosthetic valve IE, infection with Coagulase-negative staphylococci, increased duration of preoperative antibiotic therapy, shock, and the need for aortic valve replacement were all independently associated with mortality in multivariable analysis [11].

9. Prophylactic management

Medical procedures, including dental care, cardiac surgery, catheter interventions, and other non-cardiac invasive procedures are potential causes of bacteremia in up to 46%, 18%, 20%, and 20% of IE patients with CHD [9]. And IE can often be prevented by definitive repair of CHD or by reduction of bacteremia [3]. But in 2007, AHA revised the recommendation of antibiotics prophylactic guidelines to restrict preprocedural antibiotics to a few cardiac conditions that remain at higher risk for adverse outcomes related to IE [45]. And the guidelines on IE prophylaxis from international cardiology societies in 2008/2009 were greatly simplified and resulted in a drastic reduction in and limitation of cardiac diseases and procedures in which IE prophylaxis is indicated [46]. AHA guideline defines these specific cardiac conditions as follows: Prosthetic cardiac valve or prosthetic material used for cardiac valve repair, previous IE, unrepaired CHD with/without palliative shunts and conduits, completely repaired CHD with prosthetic material or device whether implanted by surgery or catheter intervention during first 6 months after the procedure, repaired CHD with residual defects at the site or adjacent to the site of a prosthetic patch or prosthetic device [45]. And ESC guidelines recommended IE prophylaxis for the patients with untreated cyanotic CHD and those with CHD who have postoperative palliative shunts, conduits, or other prostheses. After surgical repair with no residual defects, the Task Force recommends prophylaxis for the first 6 months after the procedure until endothelialization of the prosthetic material has occurred [39]. But according to the study among pediatric cardiologists, more than half of the participants (56%) do not follow the current guidelines in certain conditions such as rheumatic heart disease, Fontan palliation without fenestration, and the Ross procedure [47]. There has never been a randomized, prospective study in patients with CHD to determine whether prophylactic antibiotics provide protection against.

IE during bacteremia-inducing procedures [3]. Given the prognosis, morbidity, and excessive cost of management of IE, appropriate prophylactic strategy for prevention of IE related to CHD should be established based on much more robust data and substantial evidence. And it is emphasized that good oral hygiene, prevention of oral disease, and skin hygiene are principal factor to prevent IE [3, 4, 32].

Conflict of interest

The authors declare no conflict of interest.

Author details

Naomi Nakagawa
Department of Pediatric Cardiology, Hiroshima City Hospital, Hiroshima, Japan

*Address all correspondence to: polonekogorogoro@dream.com

References

[1] Day MD, Gauvreau K, Shulman S, Newburger JW. Characteristics of children hospitalized with endocarditis. Circulation. 2009;**119**(6):865-870

[2] Ferrieri P, Gewitz MH, Gerber MA, Newburger JW, Dajani AS, Shulman ST, et al. Unique features of infective endocarditis in childhood. Circulation. 2002;**105**(17):2115-2126

[3] Gewitz M. Infective endocarditis and prevention. In: Shaddy RE, Penny DJ, Feltes TF, Cetta F, Mital S, editors. Heart Disease in Infants, Children, and Adolescents. Including the Fetus and Young Adult. Philadelphia: Wolters Kulwer; 2022. pp. 1407-1419

[4] Baltimore RS, Gewitz M, Baddour LM, Beerman LB, Jackson MA, Lockhart PB, et al. Infective Endocarditis in childhood: 2015 update. Circulation. 2015;**105**(17):1487-1515

[5] Rosenthal LB, Feja KN, Levasseur SM, Alba LR, Gersony W, Saiman L. The changing epidemiology of pediatric endocarditis at a children's hospital over seven decades. Pediatric Cardiology. 2010;**31**(6):813-820

[6] Weber R, Berger C, Balmer C, Kretschmar O, Bauersfeld U, Pretre R, et al. Interventions using foreign material to treat congenital heart disease in children increase the risk for infective endocarditis. The Pediatric Infectious Disease Journal. 2008;**27**(6):544-550

[7] Thom K, Hanslik A, Russell JL, Williams S, Sivaprakasam P, Allen U, et al. Incidence of infective endocarditis and its thromboembolic complications in a pediatric population over 30 years. International Journal of Cardiology. 2018;**252**:74-79

[8] Rushani D, Kaufman JS, Ionescu-Ittu R, Mackie AS, Pilote L, Therrien J, et al. Infective endocarditis in children with congenital heart disease: Cumulative incidence and predictors. Circulation. 2013;**128**(13):1412-1419

[9] Knirsch W, Nadal D. Infective endocarditis in congenital heart disease. European Journal of Pediatrics. 2011;**170**(9):1111-1127

[10] Eleyan L, Khan AA, Musollari G, Chandiramani AS, Shaikh S, Salha A, et al. Infective endocarditis in pediatric population. European Journal of Pediatrics. 2021;**180**(10):3089-3100

[11] Khoo B, Buratto E, Fricke TA, Gelbart B, Brizard CP, Brink J, et al. Outcomes of surgery for infective endocarditis in children: A 30-year experience. Cardiovascular Surgery. 2019;**158**(5):1399-1409

[12] Russel HM, Jhonson SL, Wurlitzer KC, Russell HM, Johnson SL, Wurlitzer KC, et al. Outcomes of surgical therapy for infective endocarditis in a pediatric population: A 21-year review. The Annals of Thoracic Surgery. 2013;**96**(1):171-174

[13] Sun LC, Lai CC, Wang CY, Wang YH, Wang JY, Hsu YL, et al. Risk factors for infective endocarditis in children with congenital heart diseases - A nationwide population-based case control study. International Journal of Cardiology. 2017;**248**:126-130

[14] Moore B, Cao J, Kotchetkova I, Celermajer DS. Incidence, predictors and outcomes of infective endocarditis in a contemporary adult congenital heart disease population. International Journal of Cardiology. 2017;**249**:161-165

[15] Verheugt CL, Uiterwaal CS, van der Velde ET, Meijboom FJ, Pieper PG, Veen G, et al. Turning 18 with congenital heart disease: Prediction of infective endocarditis based on a large population. European Heart Journal. 2011;**32**(15):1926-1934

[16] Mylonakis E, Calderwood SB. Infective endocarditis in adults. The New England Journal of Medicine. 2001;**345**(18):1318-1330

[17] Snygg-Martin U, Giang KW, Dellborg M, Robertson J, Mandalenakis Z. Cumulative incidence of infective endocarditis in patients with congenital heart disease: A nationwide, case–control study over nine decades. Clinical Infectious Diseases. 2021;**73**(8):1469-1475

[18] Mylotte D, Rushani D, Therrien J, Guo L, Liu A, Guo K, et al. Incidence, predictors, and mortality of infective endocarditis in adults with congenital heart disease without prosthetic valves. The American Journal of Cardiology. 2017;**120**(12):2278-2283

[19] Saiman L, Prince A, Gersony WM. Pediatric infective endocarditis in the modern era. The Journal of Pediatrics. 1993;**122**(6):847-853

[20] Kelchtermans J, Grossar L, Eyskens B, Cools B, Roggen M, Boshoff D, et al. Clinical characteristics of infective endocarditis in children. The Pediatric Infectious Disease Journal. 2019;**38**(5):453-458

[21] Child JS, Pegues DA, Perloff JK. Infective endocarditis and congenital heart disease. In: Perloff JK, Child JS, Aboulhosn J, editors. Congenital Heart Disease in Adults. Philadelphia: Elsevier; 2009. pp. 168-193

[22] Slesnick TC, Nugent AW, Fraser CD, Cannon BC. Images in cardiovascular medicine. Incomplete endothelialization and late development of acute bacterial endocarditis after implantation of an Amplatzer septal Occluder device. Circulation. 2008;**117**(18):e326-e327

[23] O'Donnell C, Holloway R, Tilton E, Stirling J, Finucane K, Wilson N. Infective endocarditis following Melody valve implantation: Comparison with a surgical cohort. Cardiology in the Young. 2016;**27**(2):294-301

[24] Gröning M, Tahri NB, Søndergaard L, Helvind M, Ersbøll MK, Andersen HØ. Infective endocarditis in right ventricular outflow tract conduits: A register-based comparison of homografts, Contegra grafts and Melody transcatheter valves. European Journal of Cardio-Thoracic Surgery. 2019;**56**(1):87-93

[25] Sharma A, Cote AT, Hosking MCK, Harris KC. A systematic review of infective endocarditis in patients with bovine jugular vein valves compared with other valve types. JACC. Cardiovascular Interventions. 2017;**10**(14):1449-1458

[26] Saxena A, Aggarwal N, Gupta P, Juneja R, Kothari SS, Math R. Predictor of embolic events in pediatric infective endocarditis. Indian Heart Journal. 2011;**63**(3):237-240

[27] Fosbøl EL, Park LP, Chu VH, Athan E, Delahaye F, Freiberger T, et al. The association between vegetation size and surgical treatment on 6-month mortality in left-sided infective endocarditis. European Heart Journal. 2019;**40**(27):2243-2251

[28] Yoshinaga M, Niwa K, Niwa A, Ishiwada N, Takahashi H, Echigo S, et al. Risk factors for in-hospital mortality during infective endocarditis in patients with congenital heart disease.

The American Journal of Cardiology. 2008;**101**(1):114-118

[29] Okonta KE, Adamu YB. What size of vegetation is an indication for surgery in endocarditis? Interactive Cardiovascular and Thoracic Surgery. 2012;**15**(6):1052-1056

[30] Ye XT, Buratto E, Dimitriou J, Yaftian N, Wilson A, Darby J, et al. Right-sided infective endocarditis: The importance of vegetation size. Heart, Lung & Circulation. 2021;**30**(5):741-750

[31] Lalani T, Kanafani ZA, Chu VH, Moore L, Corey GR, Pappas P, et al. Prosthetic valve endocarditis due to coagulase-negative staphylococci: Findings from the International Collaboration on Endocarditis Merged Database. European Journal of Clinical Microbiology & Infectious Diseases. 2006;**25**(6):365-368

[32] Cox DA, Tani LY. Pediatric infective endocarditis: A clinical update. Pediatric Clinics of North America. 2020;**67**(5):875-888

[33] Wong PC. Additional applications of transesophageal echocardiography. In: Wong PC, Miller-Hance WC, editors. Transesophageal Echocardiography for Congenital Heart Disease. London: Springer; 2014. pp. 399-436

[34] Ohara T. Diagnostic strategy for infective endocarditis in patients with adult congenital heart disease. Circulation Journal. 2021;**85**(9):1514-1516

[35] Feuchtner GM, Stolzmann P, Dichtl W, Schertler T, Bonatti J, Scheffel H, et al. Multislice computed tomography in infective endocarditis: Comparison with transesophageal echocardiography and intraoperative findings. Journal of the American College of Cardiology. 2009;**53**(5):436-444

[36] Erba PA, Pizzi MN, Roque A, Salaun E, Lancellotti P, Tornos P, et al. Multimodality imaging in infective endocarditis: An imaging team within the endocarditis team. Circulation. 2019;**140**(21):1753-1765

[37] Duval X, Le Moing V, Tubiana S, Esposito-Farèse M, Ilic-Habensus E, Leclercq F, et al. Impact of systematic whole-body 18F-fluorodeoxyglucose PET/CT on the management of patients suspected of infective endocarditis: The prospective multicenter TEPvENDO study. Clinical Infectious Diseases. 2021;**73**(3):393-403

[38] Baddour LM, Wilson WR, Bayer AS, Fowler VG, Tleyjeh IM, Rybak MJ, et al. Infective endocarditis in adults: Diagnosis, antimicrobial therapy, and management of complications: A scientific statement for healthcare professionals from the american heart association. Circulation. 2015;**132**(15):1435-1486

[39] Habib G, Lancellotti P, Antunes MJ, Bongiorni MG, Casalta JP, Del Zotti F, et al. 2015 ESC guidelines for the management of infective endocarditis: The task force for the management of infective endocarditis of the European Society of Cardiology (ESC). Endorsed by: European Association for Cardio-Thoracic Surgery (EACTS), the European Association of Nuclear Medicine (EANM). European Heart Journal. 2015;**36**(44):3075-3128

[40] Kang DH, Kim YH, Kim SH, Sun BJ, Kim DH, Yun SC, et al. Early surgery versus conventional treatment for infective endocarditis. The New England Journal of Medicine. 2012;**366**(26):2466-2473

[41] Hubert S, Thuny F, Resseguier N, Giorgi R, Tribouilloy C, Dolley YL, et al. Prediction of symptomatic embolism

in infective endocarditis: Construction and validation of a risk. Journal of the American College of Cardiology. 2013;**62**(15):1384-1392

[42] Dickeman SA, Abrutyn E, Barsic B, Emilio Bouza E, Cecchi E, Moreno A, et al. The relationship between the initiation of antimicrobial therapy and the incidence of stroke in infective endocarditis: An analysis from the ICE Prospective Cohort Study (ICE-PCS). American Heart Journal. 2007;**154**(6):1086-1094

[43] Thuny F, DiSalvo G, Belliard O, Avierinos JF, Pergola V, Rosenberg V, et al. Risk of embolism and death in infective endocarditis: Prognostic value of echocardiography: A prospective multicenter study. Circulation. 2005;**112**(1):69-75

[44] Hickey EJ, Jung G, Manlhiot C, Hickey EJ, Jung G, Manlhiot C, et al. Infective endocarditis in children: Native valve preservation is frequently possible despite advanced clinical disease. The European Journal of Cardio-Thoracic Surgery. 2009;**35**(1):130-135

[45] Wilson W, Taubert KA, Gewitz M, Lockhart PB, Baddour LM, Levison M, et al. Prevention of infective endocarditis: Guidelines from the American Heart Association: A guideline from the American Heart Association Rheumatic Fever, Endocarditis, and Kawasaki Disease Committee, Council on Cardiovascular Disease in the Young, and the Council on Clinical Cardiology, Council on Cardiovascular Surgery and Anesthesia, and the Quality of Care and Outcomes Research Interdisciplinary Working Group. Circulation. 2007;**116**(15):1736-1754

[46] Nishimura RA, Carabello BA, Faxon DP, Freed MD, Lytle BW, O'Gara PT, et al. ACC/AHA guideline update on valvular heart disease: Focused update on infective endocarditis: A report of the American College of Cardiology/American Heart Association Task Force on Practice Guidelines. Circulation. 2008;**118**(8):887-896

[47] Naik RJ, Patel NR, Wang M, Shah NC. Endocarditis prophylaxis: Current practice trend among pediatric cardiologists: Are we following the 2007 guidelines? Cardiology in the Young. 2016;**26**(6):1176-1182

Chapter 6

Surgical Treatment of Infective Endocarditis

Sudeep Das De, Sanjeet Singh Avtaar Singh, Ahmed Al-Adhami and Nawwar Al-Attar

Abstract

Infective endocarditis carries a heavy disease burden with a high in-patient mortality. Surgery is the mainstay of treatment in 50% of patients diagnosed with infective endocarditis. Surgery for infective endocarditis can be challenging; a detailed understanding of surgical anatomy is essential and several fundamental principles need to be taken into consideration including optimal timing, radical debridement, decision to repair versus replace as well as the optimal choice for reconstruction. Outcomes of surgery depend on several factors including patient characteristics, the valve (s) involved, the virulence of the organism, and the extent of invasion of the infective process. Despite recent advances in treatment and improved outcomes, there remains areas for potential research including the ideal valve prosthesis/substitute and the optimal material for reconstruction. In this chapter, we will discuss the technical challenges and pitfalls in the surgical treatment of infective endocarditis, the predictors of outcome as well as novel strategies in treatment.

Keywords: endocarditis, prosthesis, surgery, repair, reconstruction

1. Introduction

The incidence of infective endocarditis is approximately 3–10 cases per 100, 000 per year and is more common in males and in the elderly. It is associated with a heavy disease burden with an in-hospital mortality ranging from 20 to 30% [1]. In native valve endocarditis (NVE), left sided heart valves are more commonly affected with right sided involvement in 5–10% of patients [2]. Surgery remains the mainstay of treatment in 50% of patients diagnosed with infective endocarditis.

2. Classification

Infective endocarditis can be classified into four groups: (1) Native valve endocarditis (NVE) (2) Prosthetic valve endocarditis (PVE) (3) Intravenous drug abuse (IVDA) infective endocarditis and (4) nosocomial infective endocarditis. The microbiology varies depending on the type of endocarditis. In community acquired IE, the most prevalent organism is Streptococcus viridians, whereas nosocomial

IE is more commonly caused by *Staphylococcus Aureus*. Native valve endocarditis of the tricuspid valve is predominantly seen in cases of IVDA with the main organism being Staphylococcus Aureus [2, 3]. Prosthetic valve endocarditis (PVE) cases that occur within the first year after surgery are considered early and cases that occur after 1 year are termed late. The offending organism in early PVE is commonly Staphylococcus Epidermis and Staphylococcus Aureus. Microbiology in late PVE is similar to native IE with Streptococcus viridians and Staphylococcus Aureus being the prevalent organism. Infective endocarditis can be further classified temporally with acute endocarditis being caused by more virulent organisms such as Staphylococcus Aureus and presenting with severe sepsis and rapid destruction of the valve and surrounding structures. Subacute endocarditis is caused by less virulent organisms such as viridians group Streptococcus and has a more indolent nature with a prolonged clinical course.

3. Pathophysiology of infective endocarditis

Infective endocarditis results from (1) Disruption of the valvular endocardial surface resulting in turbulent flow and (2) Adherence of blood bourne micro-organisms typically bacteria to the damaged endocardial surface. Endocardial damage occurs in degenerative calcific disease, rheumatic heart disease, congenital heart disease and from iatrogenic causes such as cardiac catheterization. Common causes of bacteraemia include intravenous drug abuse, long term indwelling catheters and invasive medical procedures. Complications of infective endocarditis can be from embolic phenomena including a stroke, kidney and splenic infarcts or due to direct invasion of surrounding structures resulting in problems such as paravalvular abscesses, conduction system pathology and fistulae.

4. Diagnosis, initial treatment and indications for surgery

The diagnosis of infective endocarditis is made with the modified Duke criteria [4]. A high index of suspicion is needed in cases where cultures are negative. This can occur in up to 2–7% of cases [5, 6] and is most commonly caused by premature administration of antimicrobial therapy prior to taking blood cultures, and infection with fastidious bacteria or fungi. Once blood cultures have been taken, the first line of treatment is aggressive broad spectrum antibiotics administered empirically, followed by surveillance blood cultures and serial transthoracic echocardiograms. In the recently published Partial Oral Treatment of Endocarditis (POET) trial [7], it was demonstrated that in patients with left-sided infective endocarditis from certain specified organisms, partial oral antibiotic treatment after initial intravenous treatment was non-inferior to treatment with only intravenous antibiotics. This study however has several limitations with regards to the generalisability of the findings to the general population. Firstly, only patients with left sided endocarditis caused by strep species, *E. faecalis*, *S. aureus* or coag-neg staph were included. These organisms represent 70–75% of all cases of infective endocarditis. Patients with Methicillin resistant Staph aureus (MRSA) endocarditis were not included and there were very few intravenous drug users in the study. Highly compliant patients were selected and in the outpatient oral antibiotic therapy group, patients were followed up 2 to 3 times per week and this may not reflect real world clinical practice. From a surgical perspective, there is a risk that in patients on oral antibiotic therapy being followed up in the community, the sequelae of the disease process which may necessitate surgery may be missed, leading to a higher morbidity and mortality. An inpatient setting may allow more active surveillance of the patients with serial transthoracic echocardiograms and blood tests.

The indications for surgery are in line with the American College of Cardiology (ACC)/American Heart Association (AHA) or European Society of Cardiology (ESC) guidelines [8, 9]. In general, surgery is indicated when there is heart failure, worsening sepsis despite optimal antimicrobial therapy, a high embolic risk associated with large, mobile vegetations, perivalvular abscess, and virulent causative organisms such as *S. Aureus* and fungal endocarditis. Prosthetic valve endocarditis usually requires surgical treatment.

5. Pre-operative investigations

The first line of investigation in infective endocarditis is transthoracic echocardiogram (TTE) which has a sensitivity of approximately 25% in cases where the vegetation size is less than 5 mm and 70% where the vegetation size is 6-10 mm. Trans-oesophageal echocardiography (TOE) has a sensitivity and specificity of 95 and 90%, respectively [10]. TOE is the preferred investigation in cases of prosthetic valve endocarditis and where intracardiac complications such as abscesses and fistulae are suspected. At our institution, we perform a Positron Emission Tomography/Computed Tomography (PET-CT) when there is diagnostic difficulty in cases of prosthetic valve endocarditis. When there is suspected embolic phenomena in the visceral organs, a CT Abdomen/Pelvis should be performed. When there is evidence of neurological complications, a CT and/or MRI brain is needed to detect embolic infarcts or less often a haemorrhage. Haemorrhages are associated with a higher likelihood of mycotic aneurysms and further evaluation is needed if this is suspected. In non-emergency cases, patients above 40 years of age with cardiovascular risk factors should have coronary angiography to exclude coronary artery disease. If there is a large aortic valve vegetation, however this should be avoided as there is a risk of dislodging the debris. An alternative is CT Coronary angiography; however both these investigations are associated with contrast related renal toxicity and the risks have to be evaluated.

6. Surgical principles

In general, patients undergoing urgent or emergency surgery for IE tend to be unwell, septic, coagulopathic and fluid overloaded. Pre-operatively it is essential to have blood products including platelets, fresh frozen plasma, cryoprecipitate and anti-fibrinolytic agents (especially in reoperations) available. In addition, intra-operative TOE is important in all cases of IE. Fluid overload can be addressed intraoperatively by filtration on cardiopulmonary bypass. Good exposure of the operative field is needed and we recommend a full median sternotomy in all cases. Due to many patients being in heart failure and the potential for operations to be complex and lengthy, careful attention needs to be given to myocardial protection. In addition to routine antegrade cardioplegia, in cases of severe aortic regurgitation and large aortic valve vegetations which may obstruct the coronary ostia, we administer retrograde cardioplegia.

There are also several specific fundamental principles in infective endocarditis surgery, which include: (1) Optimal timing, (2) Radical debridement, (3) Repair versus replacement strategy, (4) Optimal choice of prosthesis/material for reconstruction and 5) Avoidance of contamination of the surgical field.

6.1 Optimal timing

Optimal timing of surgery for infective endocarditis remains a challenging decision for cardiac surgeons. The benefits of delaying surgery to allow adequate antibiotic therapy and time for optimising the patients' needs to be balanced with the risks of further haemodynamic deterioration and septic emboli during the waiting period. In general, once any of the indication for surgery outlined above are presented, early surgery is recommended [11]. An exception to this is if there any neurological complications. Ischaemic embolic events are more common in haemorrhagic strokes, with north associated with a high morbidity and mortality [12, 13]. In ischaemic strokes, there is a risk of haemorrhagic conversion with systemic heparinization and cardiopulmonary bypass. It is recommended that in cases of ischaemic stroke and haemorrhagic stroke, surgery should be delayed for 2 weeks and 4 weeks respectively. Ultimately, clinical judgement should be exercised in each case for the optimal timing of surgery.

6.2 Radical debridement

It is imperative to ensure radical debridement of all infected and necrotic tissue prior to reconstruction to minimise the risk of recurrence. A thorough knowledge of surgical anatomy, especially with regards to the aortic root, the left ventricular outflow tract, intra-ventricular septum and the aorto-mitral continuity is needed to perform a safe and adequate debridement followed by reconstruction.

6.3 Repair versus replacement strategy

In clinical practice, most patients with infective endocarditis undergo valve replacement. A repair strategy is recommended if possible after the primary goal of radical debridement is achieved and there is adequate tissue remaining. This is usually more commonly the case in mitral valve endocarditis. A repair strategy avoids the need for long-term anticoagulation when compared to mechanical valves, limits the amount of prosthetic material and hence recurrence and it is also well established in the mitral position that repair offers better long term survival compared to replacement [14].

6.4 Choice of prosthesis/material for reconstruction

The choice of prosthesis should be in line with current guidelines depending on the patients age, comorbidities, compliance and presence of any contra-indications to anticoagulation. There is no evidence the suggest any difference in outcomes between biological and mechanical valve prostheses in the setting of active infective endocarditis [15, 16]. If there is limited valve leaflet/annular destruction, autologous pericardial patches can be used. In cases of more extensive destruction, a bovine pericardial patch can be used. If there is significant aortic root destruction, an aortic homograft can be used for reconstruction. We will discuss these options in further detail in the following sections.

6.5 Avoidance of contamination of the surgical field

Once debridement has been completed, it is important to ensure that there is minimal further contamination of the surgical field prior to reconstruction. Instruments used for debridement, drapes, suction and surgical gloves should be changed before proceeding.

7. Native valve endocarditis

7.1 Aortic valve

In native aortic valve endocarditis, direct local complications include destruction of the aortic annulus, formation of annular abscesses, conduction tissue pathology, and fistulae. Intra-operatively, we avoid manipulation of the heart prior to applying the aortic cross clamp and arresting the heart to avoid the risk of the aortic vegetations dislodging. A transverse autotomy is performed to expose the aortic valve. If there is annular destruction towards the aorto-mitral continuity an oblique aortotomy towards the middle of the non-coronary cusp can be performed.

If there is a small area of leaflet perforation, the valve can be repaired using autologous pericardium. In most cases the valve is excised and if the annulus is involved, complete debridement of the infected tissue is needed. The defect is then reconstructed prior to implantation of the prosthetic valve. If the defect is small, autologous pericardium is used and for larger defects bovine pericardium is an alternative. If there is significant destruction of the annulus with discontinuity of the ventriculo-aortic junction, an reconstruction with an aortic homograft is the treatment of choice [17, 18]. The size of the the homograft is usually 2-3 mm less than the diameter of the native annulus. In cases where the aorto-mitral continuity is involved, the anterior leaflet of the mitral valve from the homograft can be used for reconstruction of the disruption. The use of freestyle aortic root replacements [19] and the Ross procedure [20] has also been reported in younger patients in extensive infective endocarditis of the aortic root.

7.2 Mitral valve

In native mitral valve endocarditis, the most common site of vegetations is on the leaflets near the annulus on the atrial side. They can however involve any part of the mitral valve apparatus. In severe cases, there is destruction of the atrioventricular junction with abscess formation. In our standard practice, we perform a median sternotomy, institute bi-caval cannulation and approach the mitral valve either via Sondergaard's groove or a trans-septal approach. If there is limited involvement of the leaflet tissue, repair can be attempted after debridement. Perforations of the anterior and posterior leaflets can be repaired using an autologous pericardial patch. A frequently involved region is the P2 region of the posterior leaflet. Standard principles of mitral valve repair apply when approaching repair in the setting of infective endocarditis. A triangular resection followed by closure is performed or if a wider region of P2 is involved a quadrangular resection followed by a slideplasty of the remaining tissue. An annuloplasty ring is then secured. Whenever possible we try to avoid added prosthetic material such as neochordae when attempting repair. More often, there is limited native tissue post debridement and we proceed to mitral valve replacement. In more severe cases where there is annular destruction, the annulus has to be reconstructed. There are two approaches to annular reconstruction described by Carpentier and David.

In technique described by Carpentier [21], figure of eight sutures are applied directly to approximate the separation of the atrioventricular groove. Valve sutures with a large needle are then placed around this suture line. This technique is not commonly used and is reserved only in cases of very narrow atrioventricular defects. In the more commonly used technique described by David [22], a semi-circular pericardial patch is fashioned with one end secured to the endocardium of the ventricle and the other end to the left atrium. The patch should be larger than the defect size to avoid any tension. The mitral valve prosthesis is then secured with pledgeted sutures with part of it anchored onto the patch.

7.3 Tricuspid valve

Our approach to the tricuspid valve is via median sternotomy and bicaval cannulation with snaring of the cavae. Most surgeons at our institution arrest the heart to perform the operation. The advantage of this is a bloodless field as well as the aorta being collapsed and the aortic valve leaflets less prone to injury during the tricuspid valve procedure. In very sick patients however, the procedure can be done on a beating heart, with the additional advantage of observing any conduction defects during the operation.

In native tricuspid valve endocarditis there are three options for treatment: (1) Valvectomy, (2) Repair/Reconstruction and (3) Replacement.

When there is severe involvement of the leaflets, complete excision of the tricuspid valve can be performed and a second stage procedure can be done following aggressive antiobiotic therapy and treating the drug dependence of the patient. This can only be done if the pulmonary pressures are not high [23]. In practice however this is seldom done, and 20% of patient will develop right heart failure [24, 25]. When there is limited infection, there are several repair/reconstructive options. These include the use of pericardial patches, excision of the posterior leaflet and biscuspidization of the tricuspid valve, slideplasty and the use of neochordae [26, 27]. The reconstruction can be reinforced with an annuloplasty ring.

Several studies have shown no difference between biological and mechanical valves in the tricuspid position [28, 29]. Biological valves in the tricuspid position have also demonstrated longer durability compared those in the mitral position [30]. In addition, mechanical valves in the tricuspid position require higher INR values. For these reasons, in our clinical practice we use a mitral bioprosthesis for tricuspid valve replacement (TVR). Following TVR, we secure permanent epicardial pacing leads.

8. Prosthetic valve endocarditis

Prosthetic valve endocarditis (PVE) is more common in the aortic than in the mitral position due to more mitral valve repair cases and less prosthetic material. PVE is classified as early if it occurs within 1 year post-operatively and late if it occurs after that. The incidence of early PVE is 1% per year [31]. Early PVE is associated with intra-operative contamination. Risk factors include native valve endocarditis, longer cardiopulmonary bypass times, and long term indwelling lines and catheters. The incidence of late PVE is 0.5 to 1% per year [32, 33]. Late PVE is usually attributed to hospital-acquired infections and is seen in patients with long-term comorbidities who require frequent admissions for procedures such as haemodialysis and also in patients who are immunosuppressed. In earlyPVE, the interface between the sewing ring and annulus is usually involved resulting in valve dehiscence and a para-valvular leak. Compared to native valve endocarditis (NVE), PVE more commonly results in abscess formation involving the intraventricular septum causing conduction blocks, as well as development pseudoaneurysms. The treatment of PVE is more aggressive and surgery is usually the definitive treatment for PVE. In severe cases, PVE may extend into intervalvlular fibrosa and require replacement of both aortic and mitral valves. This is less common in native valve endocarditis. In these cases, an extended transseptal approach can be performed for improved exposure to both valves. A bovine pericardial patch can be used to reconstruct the intervalvular fibrosa. The mitral valve is secured to the annulus posteriorly, medially and laterally. The superior part of the mitral sewing ring is secured to the patch which can also be used to cover the left atrium. Once the mitral valve prosthesis is secured, the aortic valve prosthesis is then secured partly to the healthy annulus and to the patch. Attention must be given to the angle between the aortic and mitral valve prostheses to be similar to the normal aorto-mitral angle. As mentioned previously, an aortic homograft can also be used. The aorto-mitral curtain of the homograft can be used to reconstruct the native anterior mitral valve leaflet. If there is extensive damage to the native mitral valve, the mitral valve prosthesis can be secured to the intervalvular fibrosa of the homograft [17, 18].

9. Results

The results of surgery for infective endocarditis depend on several factors including patient charactersitics, the valve(s) involved, the virulence of the organism, the extent of invasion of the infective process. Generally, prosthetic valve endocarditis has a worse prognosis than native valve endocarditis [34, 35] and nosocomial infections are also associated with a poorer outcome compared to community-acquired infections [36]. In cases of isolated simple native aortic valve endocarditis, the operative mortality is less than 10% whereas more complex cases and prosthetic valve endocarditis is associated with a higher mortality [37–39]. Recent advances in operative techniques have however yielded excellent results with comparable outcomes in native versus prosthetic valve endocarditis as well as simple endocarditis compared to more invasive disease [40].

Overall, the results for mitral valve endocarditis tends to be worse compared to aortic valve endocarditis, and this is especially the case in more invasive disease. This is likely explained by the fact that it is more difficult to debride and drain the the atrioventricular groove [22]. In addition, there is currently no equivalent to the aortic homograft in the mitral position as a viable reconstructive option [41].

Mitral valve repair has shown excellent results when compared to mitral valve replacement in IE with lower in-hospital mortality as well as better overall and infection free survival [42]. This can be attributed to the fact that patients in whom mitral valve repair is feasible tend to have less invasive disease and are generally systemically better, there is less prosthetic material used, and left ventricular function is preserved with mitral valve repair.

Native tricuspid valve repair and replacement have excellent results, with repair recommended whenever feasible [28, 43]. The outcome is also dependent on patient rehabilitation and avoidance of drug dependence.

Concomitant aortic and mitral valve endocarditis is associated with a worse prognosis when compared to single valve endocarditis [40]. Similarly, concomitant right and left sided endocarditis has a worse outcome than isolated right sided endocarditis [44].

Overall the long term survival following surgery for endocarditis is reported as between 50 and 60% at 15 years. There is also no difference in survival or recurrence rates between bioprosthetic and mechanical valves [16, 34].

10. Further development

Despite the recent advances in the treatment of infective endocarditis, there remains challenges including optimal penetration of antibiotic therapy, and the ideal material or prosthesis for reconstruction. Several novel approaches have been described in pre-clinical models to tackle the problem of biofilm formation in infective endocarditis. These include non-antibiotic strategies such as the administration of anti-thrombotic agents, hyperbaric oxygen therapy, and agents which potentially disrupt the gene regulation of bacteria during biofilm formation [45]. The use of novel extra-cellular matrix patches for mitral valve as well as tricuspid valve reconstruction has also been reported [46, 47]. Allograft mitral valve replacement has also been reported in severe aortic and mitral valve endocarditis as well as in isolated tricuspid valve endocarditis [41, 48, 49]. Another area of ongoing research is the development of bioengineered valves as a viable prosthesis in the setting of infective endocarditis with the potential of avoiding biofilm formation and recurrence of infection and long term durability [50].

11. Conclusions

The surgical treatment of infective endocarditis can be challenging. A thorough understanding of surgical anatomy is essential and several fundamental principles should be taken into consideration including optimal timing, radical debridement, decision to repair versus replace as well as the optimal choice for reconstruction. The results for infective endocarditis have improved with reports of similar outcomes between simple and more invasive endocarditis. There are potential areas for further research including developing the ideal prosthesis/substitute as well as the optimal material for reconstruction.

Conflict of interest

The authors declare no conflict of interest.

Author details

Sudeep Das De[1*], Sanjeet Singh Avtaar Singh[1,2,3], Ahmed Al-Adhami[1,2] and Nawwar Al-Attar[1,2]

1 Department of Cardiothoracic Surgery, Golden Jubilee National Hospital, Glasgow, UK

2 Institute of Cardiovascular and Medical Sciences, University of Glasgow, Glasgow, UK

3 Department of Cardiothoracic Surgery, Royal Infirmary of Edinburgh, Edinburgh, UK

*Address all correspondence to: sdasde@gmail.com

References

[1] Prendergast BD. The changing face of infective endocarditis. Heart. 2006;**92**(7):879-885

[2] Moss R, Munt B. Injection drug use and right sided endocarditis. Heart. 2003;**89**(5):577-581

[3] Fowler VG Jr, Miro JM, Hoen B, Cabell CH, Abrutyn E, Rubinstein E, et al. Staphylococcus aureus endocarditis: A consequence of medical progress. Journal of the American Medical Association. 2005;**293**(24):3012-3021

[4] Durack DT, Lukes AS, Bright DK. New criteria for diagnosis of infective endocarditis: Utilization of specific echocardiographic findings. Duke Endocarditis Service. American Journal of Medicine. 1994;**96**(3):200-209

[5] Lamas CC, Eykyn SJ. Blood culture negative endocarditis: Analysis of 63 cases presenting over 25 years. Heart. 2003;**89**(3):258-262

[6] Werner M, Andersson R, Olaison L, Hogevik H. A clinical study of culture-negative endocarditis. Medicine (Baltimore). 2003;**82**(4):263-273

[7] Iversen K, Ihlemann N, Gill SU, Madsen T, Elming H, Jensen KT, et al. Partial Oral versus intravenous antibiotic treatment of endocarditis. The New England Journal of Medicine. 2019;**380**(5):415-424

[8] Bonow RO, Carabello BA, Kanu C, de Leon AC Jr, Faxon DP, Freed MD, et al. ACC/AHA 2006 guidelines for the management of patients with valvular heart disease: A report of the American College of Cardiology/American Heart Association task force on practice guidelines (writing committee to revise the 1998 guidelines for the Management of Patients with Valvular Heart Disease): Developed in collaboration with the Society of Cardiovascular Anesthesiologists: Endorsed by the Society for Cardiovascular Angiography and Interventions and the Society of Thoracic Surgeons. Circulation 2006;**114**(5):e84-231

[9] Habib G, Lancellotti P, Antunes MJ, Bongiorni MG, Casalta JP, Del Zotti F, et al. 2015 ESC guidelines for the management of infective endocarditis: The task force for the Management of Infective Endocarditis of the European Society of Cardiology (ESC). Endorsed by: European Association for Cardio-Thoracic Surgery (EACTS), the European Association of Nuclear Medicine (EANM). European Heart Journal. 2015;**36**(44):3075-3128

[10] Daniel WG, Mügge A, Grote J, Hausmann D, Nikutta P, Laas J, et al. Comparison of transthoracic and transesophageal echocardiography for detection of abnormalities of prosthetic and bioprosthetic valves in the mitral and aortic positions. The American Journal of Cardiology. 1993;**71**(2):210-215

[11] Kang DH, Lee S, Kim YJ, Kim SH, Kim DH, Yun SC, et al. Long-term results of early surgery versus conventional treatment for infective endocarditis trial. Korean Circulation Journal. 2016;**46**(6):846-850

[12] Gillinov AM, Shah RV, Curtis WE, Stuart RS, Cameron DE, Baumgartner WA, et al. Valve replacement in patients with endocarditis and acute neurologic deficit. The Annals of Thoracic Surgery. 1996;**61**(4):1125-1129 discussion 30

[13] Matsushita K, Kuriyama Y, Sawada T, Yamaguchi T, Nagata S, Kawazoe K, et al. Hemorrhagic and ischemic cerebrovascular complications of active infective endocarditis of native valve. European Neurology. 1993;**33**(3):267-274

[14] Enriquez-Sarano M, Schaff HV, Orszulak TA, Tajik AJ, Bailey KR, Frye RL. Valve repair improves the outcome of surgery for mitral regurgitation. A multivariate analysis. Circulation. 1995;**91**(4):1022-1028

[15] Byrne JG, Rezai K, Sanchez JA, Bernstein RA, Okum E, Leacche M, et al. Surgical management of endocarditis: The society of thoracic surgeons clinical practice guideline. The Annals of Thoracic Surgery. 2011;**91**(6):2012-2019

[16] Moon MR, Miller DC, Moore KA, Oyer PE, Mitchell RS, Robbins RC, et al. Treatment of endocarditis with valve replacement: The question of tissue versus mechanical prosthesis. The Annals of Thoracic Surgery. 2001;**71**(4):1164-1171

[17] Glazier JJ, Verwilghen J, Donaldson RM, Ross DN. Treatment of complicated prosthetic aortic valve endocarditis with annular abscess formation by homograft aortic root replacement. Journal of the American College of Cardiology. 1991;**17**(5):1177-1182

[18] Yankah AC, Pasic M, Klose H, Siniawski H, Weng Y, Hetzer R. Homograft reconstruction of the aortic root for endocarditis with periannular abscess: A 17-year study. European Journal of Cardio-Thoracic Surgery. 2005;**28**(1):69-75

[19] Heinz A, Dumfarth J, Ruttmann-Ulmer E, Grimm M, Müller LC. Freestyle root replacement for complex destructive aortic valve endocarditis. The Journal of Thoracic and Cardiovascular Surgery. 2014;**147**(4):1265-1270

[20] Pettersson G, Tingleff J, Joyce FS. Treatment of aortic valve endocarditis with the Ross operation. European Journal of Cardio-Thoracic Surgery. 1998;**13**(6):678-684

[21] Carpentier AF, Pellerin M, Fuzellier JF, Relland JY. Extensive calcification of the mitral valve anulus: Pathology and surgical management. The Journal of Thoracic and Cardiovascular Surgery. 1996;**111**(4):718-729 discussion 29-30

[22] David TE, Feindel CM, Armstrong S, Sun Z. Reconstruction of the mitral anulus. A ten-year experience. The Journal of Thoracic and Cardiovascular Surgery. 1995;**110**(5):1323-1332

[23] Arbulu A, Holmes RJ, Asfaw I. Tricuspid valvulectomy without replacement. Twenty years' experience. The Journal of Thoracic and Cardiovascular Surgery. 1991;**102**(6):917-922

[24] Arbulu A, Holmes RJ, Asfaw I. Surgical treatment of intractable right-sided infective endocarditis in drug addicts: 25 years experience. The Journal of Heart Valve Disease. 1993;**2**(2):129-137 discussion 38-9

[25] Robin E, Thomas NW, Arbulu A, Ganguly SN, Magnisalis K. Hemodynamic consequences of total removal of the tricuspid valve without prosthetic replacement. The American Journal of Cardiology. 1975;**35**(4):481-486

[26] Bortolotti U, Tursi V, Fasoli G, Milano A, Frigato N, Casarotto D. Tricuspid valve endocarditis: Repair with the use of artificial chordae.

The Journal of Heart Valve Disease. 1993;**2**(5):567-570

[27] Lange R, De Simone R, Bauernschmitt R, Tanzeem A, Schmidt C, Hagl S. Tricuspid valve reconstruction, a treatment option in acute endocarditis. European Journal of Cardio-Thoracic Surgery. 1996;**10**(5):320-326

[28] Carrier M, Hébert Y, Pellerin M, Bouchard D, Perrault LP, Cartier R, et al. Tricuspid valve replacement: An analysis of 25 years of experience at a single center. The Annals of Thoracic Surgery. 2003;**75**(1):47-50

[29] Ratnatunga CP, Edwards MB, Dore CJ, Taylor KM. Tricuspid valve replacement: UK heart valve registry mid-term results comparing mechanical and biological prostheses. The Annals of Thoracic Surgery. 1998;**66**(6):1940-1947

[30] Cohen SR, Silver MA, McIntosh CL, Roberts WC. Comparison of late (62 to 140 months) degenerative changes in simultaneously implanted and explanted porcine (Hancock) bioprostheses in the tricuspid and mitral valve positions in six patients. The American Journal of Cardiology. 1984;**53**(11):1599-1602

[31] Agnihotri AK, McGiffin DC, Galbraith AJ, O'Brien MF. The prevalence of infective endocarditis after aortic valve replacement. The Journal of Thoracic and Cardiovascular Surgery. 1995;**110**(6):1708-1720 discussion 20-4

[32] Fang G, Keys TF, Gentry LO, Harris AA, Rivera N, Getz K, et al. Prosthetic valve endocarditis resulting from nosocomial bacteremia. A prospective, multicenter study. Annals of Internal Medicine. 1993;**119**(7 Pt 1): 560-567

[33] Grover FL, Cohen DJ, Oprian C, Henderson WG, Sethi G, Hammermeister KE. Determinants of the occurrence of and survival from prosthetic valve endocarditis. Experience of the veterans affairs cooperative study on Valvular heart disease. The Journal of Thoracic and Cardiovascular Surgery. 1994;**108**(2):207-214

[34] David TE, Gavra G, Feindel CM, Regesta T, Armstrong S, Maganti MD. Surgical treatment of active infective endocarditis: A continued challenge. The Journal of Thoracic and Cardiovascular Surgery. 2007;**133**(1):144-149

[35] Manne MB, Shrestha NK, Lytle BW, Nowicki ER, Blackstone E, Gordon SM, et al. Outcomes after surgical treatment of native and prosthetic valve infective endocarditis. The Annals of Thoracic Surgery. 2012;**93**(2):489-493

[36] Hoen B, Alla F, Selton-Suty C, Béguinot I, Bouvet A, Briançon S, et al. Changing profile of infective endocarditis: Results of a 1-year survey in France. Journal of the American Medical Association. 2002;**288**(1):75-81

[37] Alexiou C, Langley SM, Stafford H, Lowes JA, Livesey SA, Monro JL. Surgery for active culture-positive endocarditis: Determinants of early and late outcome. The Annals of Thoracic Surgery. 2000;**69**(5):1448-1454

[38] d'Udekem Y, David TE, Feindel CM, Armstrong S, Sun Z. Long-term results of operation for paravalvular abscess. The Annals of Thoracic Surgery. 1996;**62**(1):48-53

[39] d'Udekem Y, David TE, Feindel CM, Armstrong S, Sun Z. Long-term results of surgery for active infective endocarditis. European Journal of Cardio-Thoracic Surgery. 1997;**11**(1):46-52

[40] Hussain ST, Shrestha NK, Gordon SM, Houghtaling PL,

Blackstone EH, Pettersson GB. Residual patient, anatomic, and surgical obstacles in treating active left-sided infective endocarditis. The Journal of Thoracic and Cardiovascular Surgery. 2014;**148**(3):981-8.e4

[41] Navia JL, Al-Ruzzeh S, Gordon S, Fraser T, Agüero O, Rodríguez L. The incorporated aortomitral homograft: A new surgical option for double valve endocarditis. The Journal of Thoracic and Cardiovascular Surgery. 2010;**139**(4):1077-1081

[42] Muehrcke DD, Cosgrove DM 3rd, Lytle BW, Taylor PC, Burgar AM, Durnwald CP, et al. Is there an advantage to repairing infected mitral valves? The Annals of Thoracic Surgery. 1997;**63**(6):1718-1724

[43] Gottardi R, Bialy J, Devyatko E, Tschernich H, Czerny M, Wolner E, et al. Midterm follow-up of tricuspid valve reconstruction due to active infective endocarditis. The Annals of Thoracic Surgery. 2007;**84**(6):1943-1948

[44] Musci M, Siniawski H, Pasic M, Grauhan O, Weng Y, Meyer R, et al. Surgical treatment of right-sided active infective endocarditis with or without involvement of the left heart: 20-year single center experience. European Journal of Cardio-Thoracic Surgery. 2007;**32**(1):118-125

[45] Lerche CJ, Schwartz F, Theut M, Fosbøl EL, Iversen K, Bundgaard H, et al. Anti-biofilm approach in infective endocarditis exposes new treatment strategies for improved outcome. Frontiers in Cell and Development Biology. 2021;**9**:643335

[46] Arbona MA, David TE, David CM, Rao V. Results of mitral valve reconstruction using substitute extracellular matrix. JTCVS Tech. 2022;**16**:43-48

[47] Gerdisch MW, Boyd WD, Harlan JL, Richardson JB Jr, Flack JE 3rd, Palafox BA, et al. Early experience treating tricuspid valve endocarditis with a novel extracellular matrix cylinder reconstruction. The Journal of Thoracic and Cardiovascular Surgery. 2014;**148**(6):3042-3048

[48] Couetil JP, Argyriadis PG, Shafy A, Cohen A, Berrebi AJ, Loulmet DF, et al. Partial replacement of the tricuspid valve by mitral homografts in acute endocarditis. The Annals of Thoracic Surgery. 2002;**73**(6):1808-1812

[49] Mestres CA, Castellá M, Moreno A, Paré JC, del Rio A, Azqueta M, et al. Cryopreserved mitral homograft in the tricuspid position for infective endocarditis: A valve that can be repaired in the long-term (13 years). The Journal of Heart Valve Disease. 2006;**15**(3):389-391

[50] Bonetti A, Marchini M, Ortolani F. Ectopic mineralization in heart valves: New insights from in vivo and in vitro procalcific models and promising perspectives on noncalcifiable bioengineered valves. Journal of Thoracic Disease. 2019;**11**(5):2126-2143